To: Sergey
From: H. E. Bisalski

The Naked Truth

by

H.E. Bisalski

DORRANCE PUBLISHING CO., INC.
PITTSBURGH, PENNSYLVANIA 15222

Dorrance Publishing Co., Inc.
701 Smithfield Street
Pittsburgh, PA 15222
Visit our website at *www.dorrancebookstore.com*

ISBN: 978-1-4349-1663-1
eISBN: 978-1-4349-1677-8

The Naked Truth

"Since the mind and the soul find expression through the body, both mental and spiritual vigor are in great degree dependent upon physical strength and activity; whatever promotes physical health promotes the development of a strong mind and a well-balanced character. Without health, no one can as distinctly understand or as completely fulfill his obligations to himself, to his fellow-beings, or to his Creator. Therefore, health should be as faithfully guarded as character. A knowledge of physiology and hygiene should be the basis of all educational effort." (*Education*, p. 195)

Contents

Introduction

Today we live in a society where there is more myth than truth about the way in which to have good health. Hundreds of books have been written on how to have good health, stay fit, and enjoy life to its fullest.

Most of these books have a special diet that is promoted, and you are told that if you adhere to that diet, you will receive health and happiness.

Many of these books tout an all in one pill that if you take daily, you don't have to do anything else, including exercise. The commercials on cholesterol-lowering medications are interesting. They say, "If diet and exercise are not (enough) in keeping your cholesterol down, then try Zocor, Lipitor, or Crestor." Then the ad goes in to all of the side effects of the drug, and how you need to have your liver enzymes checked frequently—why?—because these drugs could end up killing you.

Pharmaceutical companies are a trillion-dollar business. The present administration has given these companies unprecedented protection from lawsuits to come up with new drugs to protect people from everything from the common cold to HIV. Billions of dollars have been given for research of new drugs. It is a win-win situation for the pharmaceutical companies; but, is it a win-win situation for you and me?—that is the sixty-four thousand dollar question.

Do these drug cartels (pharmaceutical companies) have your best interest at heart? Do they really want a healthier society?

If drugs could cure every disease, and we had no sick people, would there be a need for medications? Absolutely not! But, drugs can't cure every disease. And drug companies are not really concerned with making you healthy so you don't have to ingest their poisons—they are primarily interested in promoting their drugs for a huge profit.

Type 2 diabetes, one of the easiest diseases to conquer by a change in lifestyle is a billion-dollar business. The companies involved in "finding a cure for type 2 diabetes" won't find it in a new drug. It's all about lifestyle change and one of the basic lifestyle changes I recommend is after instituting an exercise program and a change to a more plant-based diet is to get off all your drug-medications.

Most people don't want to get sick, not even with the common cold; and they will take just about anything to keep from getting sick especially if a drug promises a quick fix. But, will a quick fix for the short term really be the best in the long run of life?

Most people would respond, "I don't care about later, I care about now."

We need to remember when we come down with the "common cold," that's not always a bad thing. If you don't have enough sense to slow down your pace in life a bit, your body will eventually do it for you. Most of us need more rest than we are getting; but often times when our bodies are telling our minds we need rest, we look for an over the counter quick fix in the form of some medication or drug like caffeine to pump us up and get us going.

Our bodies will continue to cry out for help and for rest and if the body doesn't receive rest, it will eventually collapse.

There are so many people on antidepressants and antipsychotic drugs that if these people did not get their daily fix, we would have a society gone postal.

I have been working in the medical field since 1977, and in that thirty-three-year span, I have seen a lot of changes; but I don't know if we are any healthier because of all the advancements in medicine.

I can still remember my parents, grandparents, and my aunt saying, "Early to bed, early to rise makes a man healthy, wealthy, and wise." At the end of this book, I will expand on this old simple, but timely adage that lived and was practiced two generations ago.

Chapter One: The Single Greatest Investment of Your Life

The single best thing you can do that will have the greatest return in the long run is staying in good health. Getting out of debt is the second most important thing you can do. And the third thing to do is move out of the cities into the country where you can grow your own food and if you want meat raise your own chickens and your own beef. And for a lot of people, if they make simple lifestyle changes, they will get out of debt quicker. We are the richest nation on earth but have the costliest healthcare system in the world.

Because our emphasis is on acute care and not on long-term preventive care, we really are not any healthier than the people in England and other places. So I don't know that we're getting that much greater care for what it is costing us. With all the changes on the horizon with the new healthcare plan revisions coming from Congress—and don't kid yourself they are coming—we may not enjoy the good medical care we have become accustomed to in the past. The money just isn't there. And you know what, I'm glad the money isn't there; because now people are searching for ways to become healthier.

Just last week, our anesthesia group received a certified letter from Medicare informing us that all anesthesia providers' reimbursement would be cut 8.5 percent. Our general surgeon also received the same letter.

In the preventive realm, we are receiving better medical care. In the technological area, the United States is unsurpassed.

But what is so sad is for all the billions of dollars we pay for the high-tech healthcare, we are not living longer, healthier lives. There is a group of people who are living longer and healthier lives. They are the Seventh-Day-Adventists. They live anywhere from eight to eleven years longer than the general population and are vibrant and active. I will come back to this group of people later.

I see people every day as patients who I administer anesthesia to and some who are from fifty to eighty years of age who are carting around oxygen tanks. I don't consider that a healthy life. And most of these patients are where they are because of lifestyle choices they have made. Living an unhealthy lifestyle may take several decades to really reveal itself. The human body and mind are an incredible masterpiece of creation; but after persistent misuse, even this beautiful work of creation will take its toll and we experience that toll in sickness and in death.

Everyone comes into this world with a suitcase full of hereditary traits that give some people a jump-start on life while others struggle with diseases that are no fault of their own. That is just life. But that is where we all begin, and that is where I'd like to begin.

When we start out in life after birth, what we are is seventy percent hereditary and thirty percent of the lifestyle our parents and grandparents have given us and the environment we have been placed in. And the lifestyle our parents give us affects us in our physical, mental, psychological, and spiritual development.

I am a firm believer that you have a responsibility to improve your DNA for the next generation, because they may inherit your DNA. You can't rewrite your DNA by yourself, but God can't do it without you.

I heard the story of a young lady, eighteen or nineteen years of age, who had been diagnosed with anorexia. Her mother, her sister, and her aunt all had anorexia. So was this a hereditary disease that was passed down and the daughter had no choice but to accept it? This young girl decided after watching her mother, sister, and aunt struggle all those years with anorexia, she wanted to make a change. She did make changes and no longer has anorexia. But the interesting thing is how the mother, sister, and aunt responded to the young girl's recovery. When the families would get together for a family reunion, the four women who had anorexia would feed on each other's negative vibrations. It is very difficult for anyone to step out and make changes if everyone around you is satisfied with mediocrity. So needless to say the mother, sister, and aunt were not very happy that the young girl had overcome anorexia. Why? Because now they would have to listen to her tell them that they, too, could overcome their anorexia. They didn't want to believe that it wasn't hereditary. They did not want to overcome anorexia. They were feeding off each other's negativism.

In modern psychiatry, we would say this person is suffering from or subject to *hypochondria*, a person who worries or talks excessively about his or her health—a hypochondriac.

I recently wanted to help a young man, thirty years old, to quit smoking. After explaining some things we could do for him, he said something that surprised me: "I like smoking. It tastes good after eating to light up a cigarette. I really don't want to quit."

The NAKED TRUTH is smoking is an acquired taste. You didn't say, "I love the taste of cigarettes" the first time you lit up—you had to acquire that taste, and it's not the taste that kept you lighting up another cigarette, it's the addiction to nicotine; but you had to first overcome the coughing and gagging you experienced when you first started smoking—a protective mechanism God placed within you.

The coughing that you experienced when you first started smoking is caused by nicotine's ability of putting to sleep the little hair-like projections called cilia that line the breathing tubes that lead to your lungs.

A friend of mine who was taking medications for high blood pressure and high cholesterol and subsequently diagnosed with adult onset diabetes told me "I can't help it. It's in my family genes. My aunt had diabetes. I just have to face the fact that I have these diseases and I will always be on medication." And yes he is still a diabetic and is taking medications for diabetes, high blood pressure, and high cholesterol. Some people just think this is a cross they must bear or it's just their lot in life; but the NAKED TRUTH is there is no cross to bear here. Get off the soapbox and stop feeling sorry for yourself. This is exactly what the pharmaceutical companies (drug cartels) would like you to believe.

Someone once said, "Heredity is the loaded gun; but lifestyle pulls the trigger." So except in extreme cases of congenital defects, changing your lifestyle can make a tremendous change in what you were given in your hereditary suitcase.

I was adopted at the age of three. After my adoptive parents took custody of me, they went to pick me up. My biological mother told them where I was. They found me atop Lookout Mountain in Chattanooga, Tennessee, where two winnows were babysitting me. My adoptive parents told me years later all my teeth were messed up. Many times instead of a bottle of milk, I would be given a bottle of coke or some other soda drink. So without some lifestyle interventions, hereditarily speaking, I was in trouble.

Right here I would like to stress how important it is to teach your children to drink water at an early age. Our children have always drank plenty of water and although at times they will choose a root beer or a sprite, most of the time they choose water. Don't feed your infants and children juices unless they are freshly squeezed. When our children were little and we had an abundance of oranges that we needed to use up, I would make some fresh squeezed O.J. And if we had other fruit that needed to be eaten up, we would make smoothies. Break up a banana, cut up an apple, peel an orange, slice up some pineapple put it all in a blender add some frozen blueberries and add a half cup or a whole cup of soymilk and you have a delicious smoothie.

If you are a young mother expecting, please breast-feed your infants. There is no better way for your little ones to get a jump-start on life than for you to breast-feed them. Provided you are eating nutritiously, breast-feeding will give your infants strong immune systems. It was actually popular in the 1800's for mothers of rich or famous families to let other women breast-feed their infants so they could tend to entertaining their guests.

That was a very big mistake because their infants would actually acquire some of the hereditary traits of the women who were breast-feeding them.

I was very fortunate to have been adopted by a Christian couple. My new mother was a registered nurse and my new father a nutritionist. They were vegetarians. They were lacto-ova vegetarians; that is, they ate eggs and drank milk. They were not vegans nor did they ever take on that change in their diet.

After being adopted, we moved from Madison, Tennessee, where my father was involved in health food research, to Hot Springs, Arkansas, and there, in 1954, my dad opened up a restaurant and health food store. It was called "Foods for Health." We sold health foods, vitamins, had a juice bar, and served a complete vegetarian meal daily. My dad would present a lecture daily and answer questions on health-related topics at the end of the lecture. Our store was large. It had an upstairs complete with bedrooms, bathrooms, living room, and office and a large porch where we and our friends would watch the parade from each year. The back of the store butted almost up to the hills of the Hot Springs National Park. My brothers and I would walk out the upstairs door cross a bridge over the alley that ran behind the storefronts where we would play for hours in the hundreds of acres of Hot Springs National Park.

We also had a home off lakeshore drive in the country where we had access to Lake Hamilton. The winters were very mild, so my three brothers and I would spend a lot of time swimming and boating in the lake.

We had fifteen acres where we raised goats. To this day, I can't tell you what kind of goats we had, but I do remember milking them often. My mother would make goat cheese and we would sell the goat cheese and the goats' milk at our store. As my father would counsel people on lifestyle changes they needed to make to be in better health, he soon discovered that many of the children's allergies were brought on or worsened by drinking cow's milk or eating dairy products. So when he introduced them to goats' milk, many times the allergies disappeared. There were some who were allergic to even goat milk, and for those, my father recommended soymilk.

So as I grew up, I observed my parents practicing good health principles. I listened to my father talk with many people in helping them begin to make good lifestyle changes. It was 1954 when my father opened the health food store. In the fifties, people overall were not really health conscious. So he was really ahead of his time. My father had a passion for helping people make lifestyle changes so they could live healthier and happier lives. I'm certain that is where my passion for helping others enjoy a healthier life came from.

In the fifties, many people smoked. Hollywood dramatized smoking and drinking. In one hand, a movie star held a cigarette or cigar and in the other hand, he had a glass of wine. It was ironic that our health food store was situated in between a candy and cigar store and a lounge. And next to the lounge was a casino.

I later found out the reason my dad chose Hot Springs for a health food store was Hot Springs was a resort city and many people came from all over the country and even from other parts of the world for the famous hot baths. For the most part, those who came were looking for a better lifestyle.

Today, with the rising cost of healthcare and the skyrocketing expense of medications, you don't have to be a rocket scientist to understand that by making some simple lifestyle changes, you can save thousands of dollars. They know healthcare is a multi-billion (trillion)-dollar business, this is why the federal government wants to control healthcare. We now have a run-away national debt in this country and not enough money to pay for it—that is why our federal government wants to control the healthcare system. Congress knows that we are in deep financial trouble and they're looking for monies from anywhere to pay for this monster debt.

Many people spend their entire lives working long hours sometimes working two jobs or at least mom and dad working full time. Why? So someday they can retire and enjoy the fruits of their labor. But so often when they finally get to retirement, their health is in the toilet. And now they begin using up their retirement to pay for expensive medical treatment and for medications in an attempt to get their health back. If only they had made some simple lifestyle changes early, they would probably have their retirement and their health intact.

When you get to the end of your life, what you are is thirty percent heredity and seventy percent lifestyle. Notice how the seventy and thirty percent figures have switched places. So it is in all of our best interest to invest in some simple lifestyle changes now because making changes later may not be an option.

Be careful about reading health books. You may die of a misprint.

—Mark Twain

So go with me as we find out how to make some simple lifestyle changes that will really change your life forever.

Chapter Two: Keep a Diary for One Week

According to the dictionary, honesty has to do with sincerity and freedom from deceit and fraud. So when you begin keeping a diary, be absolutely honest with yourself. Lay out for one week all that you do. Be sincere, and at the end of one week you will be free from deceit; you will also begin feeling better. This is why many times, people get depressed over making changes in their lifestyle for whatever reasons. Remember how you felt when someone deceived you, or just wasn't quite honest and up front with you? I bet that really bothered you—it bothers me. But think about when you have deceived yourself. Now, that is the worse deceit you can ever experience.

Take note on what you eat, when you eat, and how you eat. For instance, in the morning, what did you eat for breakfast? When did you eat breakfast? How did you eat breakfast? What I'm talking about in this last question is: Did you eat on the run or while driving to work? Did you eat fast? Did you wash your food down with coffee, tea, soda pop, or water?

Then, write down the effects of your eating or drinking. Did you experience heartburn or reflux? Did you have any other kind of indigestion? Did you get a headache? Did you feel sleepy? Did you have less energy or more energy?

These are important questions because what you eat, when you eat, and how you eat may be contributing to how you feel right after you have eaten or at the end of the day or when you get up in the morning.

Also, write down in your diary what you did after you ate breakfast, lunch, and supper. For instance, did you go directly into a stressful board meeting after eating? Did you take a walk after lunch or supper? Did you go to bed right away after eating supper? Did you watch television just before retiring for the day?

It is very important you write down what you ate between meals. Eating between meals is a very deleterious habit to have. But if you really feel you need something to eat between meals, make it a healthy snack. Some of you may be saying, "But I have to keep my metabolism going, so I eat something about every two hours and just before I go to bed." We'll discuss all that later but for now, just keep that journal.

Keep record of the time you go to bed and when you get up; and what you have to do or take or eat before you go to bed or when you first get up. Sleep (how much you get and when you get it) has everything to do with lifestyle and good health.

A diary can be a real revelation. I knew one lady who said, "I never eat sweets," but when she looked at her diary at the end of one week, she saw where she was eating more sweets than she ever had imagined. Sometimes it is a real eye opener. Don't be intimidated by your diary. It will be a great tool when you decide to make some simple lifestyle changes.

At the hospital I work in at lunch every day, they serve a variety of tasty desserts. Most of the time, the employees select one of the desserts. I'm not sure if they even think about it. It is just ingrained into the American diet to eat a piece of dessert when you finish your meal.

Studies have shown it takes about twenty-one days to form a new habit. That is true with good and bad habits. When I help people stop smoking, I encourage them to begin some new habits to replace the old habit of smoking. Believe it or not, that is how many people got addicted to smoking. I know nicotine is an addicting drug, but if you didn't continue to smoke, it couldn't have become a habit and you probably wouldn't be smoking today, if you do at all.

Many of the things we do throughout the course of a day are involuntary, or they are now habit. They started out to be a voluntary choice, but after it becomes a habit or you become addicted, it is now involuntary or in large part out of your control.

That is what keeping a diary does. It puts you back in control. So many people are out of control in their lifestyle. This will be your blueprint to victory in living a long, happy, and successful life. Changing your lifestyle oftentimes gives you more energy; and if you have more energy, you will be happier and more successful.

If you ever read someone's diaries, you'll find setbacks, discouragements, as well as resolve and determination to move forward and learn from yesterday's mistakes. Those who are able to move forward and who become successful usually have made some real changes in their lives. A man told me once that he was sick and tired of being sick and tired. He wanted something better.

If you're sick and tired of being sick and tired of your lifestyle, then stay with me, for over the next several chapters I will share with you the Naked Truth of how to change your lifestyle. There are no gimmicks, no pills, and no quick fixes; but, I guarantee you when you apply and put into practice the principles I am about to share with you into your lifestyle, you will never be the same again.

Chapter Three: The Diseases that Lifestyle Changes Can Affect (An Overview)

Over the next eight chapters, I will discuss each of these diseases that lifestyle changes can either prevent, diminish the symptoms of, or reduce the amount or dosage of medications you are taking. Less medication equals more money in your pocket. So not only do you get better physical health, you will also experience improved financial strength; and in this struggling economy, we can all use more money.

Just the other day, I was making a pre-op visit on an elderly lady going for surgery. The couple were in their seventies and very pleasant. Later that morning, the nurse told me that the husband was told by his doctor to take a medication for severe acid reflux or he may be looking at esophageal or stomach cancer sooner than later; but the husband informed the nurse his wife was also told to take the same medication. The husband said because the medication was so expensive they couldn't afford for both of them to take the medication so he opted out of taking it. Only his wife was now getting the medication. I had to turn away when I heard that story. What love that man has for his wife; and what greed in the pharmaceutical companies for not making these medications readily available and affordable for everyone especially for the elderly. But drugs are never the answer. Making simple changes in lifestyle is the key. If the husband and wife institute some changes in their lifestyle, neither one will need any of those expensive medications and will not die from acid reflux. It will disappear and so will the cost of those drug-medications.

Health depends largely on lifestyle. Many erroneously believe that inherited traits (genetic factors) are the primary factors determining their quality of life and how long they will live. For the vast majority of us, our health is primarily dependent on two factors: (1) what we put into our bodies and, (2) what we do with our bodies.

The former exercise guru Jack Lalanne was quoted as saying, "Exercise is king, nutrition is Queen, put them together and you've got a kingdom." Jack lived to the grand old age of ninety-six.

A simple word that encapsulates both of these concepts is "lifestyle." The good news is that even though we cannot change our genetics, we can change our lifestyle. Those lifestyle choices can prevent or forestall the development of diseases for which we are genetically predisposed.

Regarding the most common diseases, Dr. Lamont Murdoch of Loma Linda University School of Medicine has put it aptly: "Faulty genetics loads the gun; lifestyle pulls the trigger." You don't have to commit suicide by pulling the trigger; you and you alone decide.

I have often wondered why people take better care of their cars than they do their bodies. You wouldn't think of pouring sugar into your gas tank or into the oil reservoir in your car, into the very source that every moving part receives its lubrication making your car run well. Well, that is the very thing we do when we eat and drink the wrong things, refuse to exercise, and don't get enough sleep.

Here are some of the diseases that making some simple lifestyle changes can either reverse or reduce in terms of symptoms or complications:

- Stress
- High Blood Pressure
- Diabetes (adult onset)
- **GERD** (gastroesophageal reflux disease)

- Obesity
- Depression
- Cancer
- AIDS

Chapter Four: Stress

I put stress at the top of the list because many times, the diseases that follow in the above list are either brought on by stress or are made worse by stress. We know that some stress is a good thing. Students are under a certain amount of stress to do well in school. Employees actually accomplish more if their employer knows how to apply just enough stress to help them achieve their goals. How do you know when you have too much stress? When you start experiencing symptoms that become chronic? We all encounter symptoms, sometimes, even from healthy stress, but they don't last, they don't affect us physiologically, they don't become chronic, and the symptoms do not keep us from performing our daily activities. When stress starts to affect us physiologically or prevents us from carrying out our daily activities, then we can end up with things like high blood pressure, diabetes, obesity, M.S., depression, and cancer. But I must say that even under healthy stress some people need help in understanding how to cope.

A recent study revealed that students in high school or in college who are working while attending school, overall, have higher GPA's. You know these students are under some stress. Dave Ramsey, the financial genius who stole grandma's recipes for getting out of debt and staying debt free was asked who would you hire of these two college graduates. The one who took out loans to attend college and graduated with a 4.0 but has student loans of $60,000, or the one who worked his way through college, has no student loans, but only has a 3.5 GPA? Dave said he would hire the one with the lower GPA and who has no student loans because he had to work. What was his reasoning? The student who works while attending college and who has little or no debt when he or she graduates has learned to manage their time wisely. That goes a long way with a CEO in a company who is looking for someone to hire.

It is when too much stress is employed that it literally begins to make changes in our bodies physiologically. We all have stress in our lives, some more than others; but, it's not the stress that comes to each of us that affects us physiologically, as much as it is how we handle that stress. Many students get stressed when preparing for an exam and one of two things happens: They either do poorly or they do well. Some get diarrhea, experience stomach cramps, can't sleep, get headaches, or become nervous. Many of these symptoms end up affecting them physiologically.

If stress is not controlled, your blood pressure will start to go up. You may get headaches. You may have trouble focusing or concentrating or you can't sleep. You become irritable and begin to snap back at people. There are a myriad of symptoms associated with stress that many people attribute as symptoms to whatever disease process stress is causing; and so the doctor may prescribe a blood pressure pill because the patient comes to the doctor with high blood pressure. But many times this just may be a symptom of stress; bring the stress under control or eliminate the stress and your blood pressure goes down. Is this always the case? Absolutely not, but many times it is.

Many times when I interview patients before I administer anesthesia, I notice that their blood pressure is abnormally high that morning. And I usually ask them do you have trouble with hypertension? And many times in an otherwise healthy patient they will say, "No, but every time I come to the hospital my blood pressure goes up." And even though that is not usually a bad thing, it demonstrates how stress affects us physiologically.

Recently, I spoke to a graduating class of anesthesia students. I am president of the alumni association at MTSA (Middle Tennessee School of Anesthesia) and I was asked to welcome the new class of seventy-two as official alumni. Graduation was over, they had received their diplomas, awards had been given, and I knew they did not want to listen to me go on for any great length of time. So I shared with them a story I had heard recently. "Two men who were brothers living in the same town were very evil, but they also were extremely rich. They belonged to the same church and from the outside, they were thought of as good Christians. One day, one of the brothers up and died very suddenly. His death had not been anticipated. The other brother went to their pastor and with a check in his hand said, 'I would like to give a large donation to the church, but with one condition.' The pastor asked what that condition might be. The brother said, 'When you perform my brother's funeral, you must say he was a saint.' The pastor thought for a minute and responded, 'okay....' He took the check and promptly deposited it in the church's bank account. A few days later, when they had the funeral service, the pastor got up and pointing at the casket said, "This was a very wicked man. He lied, he stole, he cheated, and he hurt a lot of people." After going on like this for a few minutes, the pastor finally said, "but compared to his brother, he was a saint."

You should have seen those graduates' faces after that story. They were happy and just for a moment they had no cares or as the Australians say, "No worries!" Just minutes before that, I had shaken each of their hands and given them an alumni pen. Some had smiles, but others were somber and just wanted the graduation to be over. But after the story, there was not one face that didn't have a smile. That's because just for a moment their hearts were filled with joy.

Now I hope that made you laugh. At that graduation, my closing comments were, "Enjoy life, have fun, laugh often, thank you, God bless you and goodnight." Words are powerful. They can bring hope, joy, happiness, and healing or they can bring sadness, sorrow, and depression, or disease.

After relating that story to the graduates, my challenge to them was "Don't let anything or anyone steal that joy I see in your faces right now."

Someone once said that adults laugh about three-four times a day, while children laugh 300-400 times a day. Now I don't know how you measure a laugh, but that is a considerable difference. I know part of the reason why children laugh more often than adults do is because they don't yet have the stress we have. There certainly are exceptions to the rule. I've met some children who I hardly ever heard laugh, but oftentimes that is because they have been hurt deeply. And although that breaks my heart, I will not and cannot let their hurt steal my joy. I want to have joy so I can share that joy with those kids and adults who are hurting.

Abraham Lincoln said, "You are as happy as you choose to be." Isn't that great! You are the one who decides how happy you will be—no one else. You might be thinking, "Well, only God can bring happiness to a person's life." I agree, but you are the only one who can decide to receive it.

There is an old song I sang in my Sabbath school class as a young boy: "Count your blessings, name them one by one, count your blessings see what God hath done." I loved that song then and I love it now and I still sing it. A song in the heart is better than a bur in the saddle. Many people look like they have a bur in their saddle as they ride through life. They're always complaining, never smiling, finding fault with everybody and everything in life. What a miserable existence. But the NAKED TRUTH is they have made a choice to be unhappy and miserable. We can't let the circumstances in our lives take away our joy. When we let something or someone steal our joy, we also let them take away our happiness.

I just want to take a moment right here to interject something that is a growing concern of mine and should be for every caring parent. With all the promiscuity, the promiscuous sexual behavior especially of our youth, the public schools handing out birth control paraphernalia like condoms and birth control pills and by law the kids don't have to have parental approval in some places, is it any wonder our society is spiraling down to such decadence? *Some historians hold that the fall of Rome can be attributed to internal decadence.* I hear all the time that everyone needs to practice safe sex. The only safe sex is sacred sex. What is sacred sex? It is a union between a man and a woman who are married.

Many young people think if they have oral or anal orgies they are not actually having sex. We can thank former President Clinton for that philosophy. But the naked truth is you don't have to have intercourse to have sex. Girls, if a guy will not stay with you unless you perform oral sex then honestly, you don't need that type of guy. Premarital sex—and especially with multiple partners—only brings regret, remorse, and heartache. When a girl enters a relationship with a guy, she is looking for love, but rarely finds it. When a guy enters a relationship with a young girl, he's looking for sex and often gets it.

One of my favorite singers who sang gospel music but who couldn't play an instrument or read music, sold more than forty-five million records in his career. He has been married for fifty-seven years, and he and his wife raised four daughters in the middle of Hollywood, California, the heart of immorality. When he gave away his four daughters to be married, they were virgins. Have you guessed who this is? That's right—Pat Boone. Well, years ago, Pat Boone and Pastor Billy Graham were scheduled to appear on the Dick Cavett program live. Neither of them knew the other was appearing at the same time. Pastor Billy Graham went on first and sometime during the interview, Dick asked Pastor Graham, "Do you really believe in not having sex unless you're married?" and, of course, Pastor Graham said, "Yes, I do." The audience broke out into a roaring laugh. Pat Boone followed Pastor Graham on the show. He was going to sing a gospel song when Dick asked him the same question. Pat responded the same as Pastor Graham, and added, "I see your audience thought Pastor Graham's answer was pretty funny, but there is one person who doesn't think that's so funny." The audience suddenly grew silent and Dick Cavett asked, "Who's that Pat" and Pat said, "Ruth." Ruth was Pastor Graham's wife.

You want to lower your stress in your life, you can begin by living a pure and chaste life. If you have already been involved with premarital sex, don't go there again until you are married legally and morally correct. You can never get your physical virginity back again once you have had premarital sex; but, I've got good news-you can become a spiritual virgin.

When we are unhappy or wear a frown on our faces, our muscles are tight; you can feel the tension in your face. But to smile and be happy, all you have to do is just relax. And the more you relax, the greater smile you wear. Remember, before the age of computers and digital cameras, we went down to Olan Mills or some other photography studio to have our pictures taken. If you had little children, you wanted to get pictures to send to grandpa and grandma that made everybody look happy. To accomplish this, a good photographer would act like a clown behind the camera to get the whole family laughing. It was great. Even the sourpusses with their scowling facial expressions were laughing at the end of the photo shoot.

But we all know it takes more than a clown once a year for family photos to make us happy and keep us laughing. A three thousand-year-old proverb found in the book of Proverbs from the Bible hasn't changed: "Laughter doeth good like a medicine." If you are going to be happy every day, you have to choose to get up on the inside. On the outside, everything may not be going your way. Your wife or your husband may be leaving you. You may have lost your job. You may have learned you have cancer. You may be losing your home through no fault of your own. These are all things that you wake up to on the outside. These are circumstances in your life that can steal your joy. Only you can determine whether these circumstances surrounding you will steal your joy. And the way you do that is to get up on the inside. No matter what is happening in your life on the outside, you have already made a choice to be happy on the inside. That old adage "Money can't buy happiness" is still true; but if you have happiness, you are rich already.

When people go to a doctor, it is usually because something is not exactly right with their body or mind. They are experiencing symptoms as the effects of some organ of their body is out of sync. They may say, "I can't sleep. I have headaches. I'm always tired. I just don't feel good." And I could go on and on of the symptoms patients tell their doctors they are experiencing. And a lot of these symptoms are the direct result of stress in their lives.

Continued untreated or wrongly treated stress will finally lead to physiological changes in the body and mind. Wrongly treated stress is when a person's symptoms' are treated with medications only, without making some simple lifestyle changes. Medications have their place in the short-term treatment while a person is instituting some simple lifestyle changes. I use medications every day in administering anesthesia for people having surgery. Although some people may have to be on medication the rest of their lives, the amount or dosage can be reduced significantly by again introducing some simple lifestyle changes.

The single greatest gift you can receive or give is health. It is the only gift that truly keeps on giving. If you don't have health, what do you have? When you come to your retirement years expecting to enjoy the fruits of your labor and you don't have good health, will you then say, "I wish I had spent more time at the office or I wish I had worked later every day." No, I don't think so.

I work with a lady in our hospital who has spent forty-four years working in surgery as a scrub tech. Her husband has been dead for several years and she lives alone. She now has high blood pressure, high cholesterol, and a myriad of other health problems. She moves slowly, just doesn't feel good, and the doctors can't seem to help her feel better. Every time she returns from a clinic or hospital, another drug has been suggested or her present medications adjusted.

We live in an allopathic society. Just give me a pill that will make me feel better, quicker, because I don't have time to slow down. I asked this scrub tech, "What would you do differently, if you could live your life over again?"

She said, "I would spend more time with my family." In all respect to the hospital she works in, her forty-four years of service will soon be forgotten after she is gone.

Is the drive to succeed keeping you under too much stress? What would you win by walking away from your present lifestyle? That is what you may have to do in changing your life style to experience good health.

In the bible, in the book of Matthew, chapter eight verses twenty-three and twenty-four, we find Jesus in a boat with His disciples on the sea in the midst of angry waters. "Now, when He got into a boat, His disciples followed Him. And suddenly a great tempest arose on the sea, so that the boat was covered with the waves. But He was asleep." How could that be? How could anyone sleep during such a stressful time as that? Most people love this story, especially the part where Jesus stands up in that storm-tossed boat and commands the winds and the waves to "be still." But it seems to me there is even a larger lesson looming here in the simple fact that He was sound asleep in a sinking boat that was taking on water, with the wind howling and the stinging rain all around Him. Christ had placed Himself in the hands of his Father, and he could sleep completely, deeply, and untroubled no matter what the commotion and fear all around him was. And although we shouldn't be asleep literally all the time when everything seems to be going down around us, we can rest and have peace while the world around us is falling apart.

There can be peace, free from stress, on the inside if we allow that transforming grace to permeate our heart and mind completely. On the outside, the storms of life may be raging. You may be going through a divorce. You may have lost a son or daughter or some close friend. You may be facing financial disaster. You may have just learned you have cancer and you only have a few months to live. Whatever the storms you're facing on the outside, on the inside you can hear those beautiful words Jesus spoke some two thousand years ago, "Peace, be still, I will never leave you or forsake you."

Frankly, I think Jesus would probably tell us that multitasking is a tool of the devil. The Creator did not make human beings to be pushed to the limit, sucked dry of every bit of energy in order for employers to increase productivity. We have a pandemic of degenerative diseases in America that are the direct result of trying to get too much out of life without putting the same investment back in. Everyone wants to win the lottery; everyone wants to get more than they pay for. At least 40 percent of Americans are on some form of entitlement-unemployment or welfare subsidy. Very soon, Jesus is coming back to tell us, "Enough is enough!"

I call it information overload. We experience it from the television, computers, cell phones, iPads, iPods, laptops, and all the other high tech gadgetry that we have; the human mind needs time to rest from all this information overload.

So how do we overcome stress? I think a better question is: How do we deal with stress in our lives?

The other day, I was taking a medical history from a forty-six-year-old female patient. She was on Zanax and some other anti-anxiety medications to help her cope with stress and anxiety in her life. I asked her how she was doing in handling stress in her life, and she smiled and said, "My doctor said if I would just divorce the stress in my life, I wouldn't need these medications."

We both laughed. I don't know of anybody that has gone through a divorce who hasn't added more stress to their life, especially if children are involved. But I do know there are times that divorce is the best solution for all parties involved.

If there is something in your life that is causing you stress and you can eliminate it, then that is where you begin. If we go back to chapter two and look over the journal that you kept, you will discover things there that are causing you stress. If you can eliminate something you find there that is causing you anxiety, then remove it.

So the first part of lowering stress in our life is to remove or eliminate anything that is in our power to remove or eliminate; if, however, you find that whatever is causing your stress you cannot at this time eliminate, then plan B begins—learning how to deal with that stress.

Plan A is eliminate stress where you can; Plan B is learn how to deal or cope with your stress.

My oldest daughter is going through a divorce, and recently she was visiting my wife and me for the weekend, which actually turned into a week and at the week's end, it all turned out for the good. They have two boys ages fourteen and twelve. At the age of thirty-eight, she now feels a need to go back to school and become a teacher, for which my wife and I applaud her. SAU (Southern Adventist University) is only ten minutes from our home where she has shown an interest to attend college. She spent the week inquiring about housing for her and her sons, and checking on student aid. SAU was most accommodating and she returned sure that things would work out if she decided to move. Her job was transferable almost immediately. Her two sons had already expressed an interest, even before the divorce issue surfaced, to go to the school that is right next to SAU.

I could see as the week wore on that she was very stressed and really struggling with a decision of moving or staying where she now was living.

About midweek after she had completed all the paperwork for grants, loans, and the usual things associated with attending college, I said to her, "The stress that you are under right now that is making you so unhappy and is stealing your joy, is not your ex-husband; no, your stress is caused by you living on the field of indecision.

I told her after she has checked everything out about going back to school at both places, to make a decision and stick to it and let the chips fall where they will.

The next morning, my daughter said, "You know, Dad, you are right (Boy, you don't hear that very often). I've been torn up on the inside because I haven't made a decision." Well, good news, she had made a decision and was happier for it.

My mother used to say, "The field of indecision is the devil's playground," and she was correct. It is better to make a wrong decision than to make no decision at all. If you do make the wrong decision, at least now you can make a change and make corrections to reset your GPS. But if you don't make a decision, you may never find your answer, and that is where a lot of unwanted stress comes from.

Former President Ronald Reagan once had an aunt who took him to a cobbler for a pair of new shoes. The cobbler asked young Reagan, "Do you want square toes or round toes?" Unable to decide, Reagan didn't answer, so the cobbler gave him a few days. Several days later, the cobbler saw Reagan on the street and asked him again what kind of toes he wanted on his shoes. Reagan still couldn't decide, so the shoemaker replied, "Well, come by in a couple of days. Your shoes will be ready." When the future president did so, he found one square-toed and one round-toed shoe! "This will teach you to never let people make decisions for you," the cobbler said to his indecisive customer. "I learned right then and there," Reagan said later, "if you don't make your own decisions, someone else will."

Kevin Carter could never escape his continent's turmoil. For a decade, the photographer captured vivid pictures of repression and strife in his native South Africa. Last year, he went to famine-racked Sudan and came upon a starving toddler stalked by a vulture. He photographed the scene—an image that won this year's Pulitzer Prize—then chased the vulture away. As the child resumed her walk to a feeding station, he lit a cigarette and wept. Last week, at thirty-three, he killed himself with carbon monoxide pumped into his pickup truck. Explained his father: "Kevin always carried around the horror of the work he did," *U.S. News and World Report*, August 8, 1994.

I want to take a moment and salute our great fighting forces in every branch of service that are in the U.S. military and every police officer and every firefighter who, in the line of duty, have to experience and see things every day that they have to live with for the rest of their lives. When you see one of these brave heroes, tell them how much you appreciate them for the protection they provide you. You'll help lower their stress and you will lower your stress by giving. Also, my heart goes out to all the family members who have lost loved ones in one of these specialties.

Oh, friends, today, if you're reading this book and are so discouraged or depressed to the point of contemplating suicide like this young man, Kevin did...—STOP! There is a way out of your gloom and darkness that seems to be all about you.

I remember years ago when traveling and getting ready to board an airplane, that the weather was gloomy, overcast with clouds, rainy, and I was feeling a little down; I muttered to myself, "Won't the sun ever shine to drive these clouds away?" Still feeling that way sitting in my seat in the airplane, the pilot's voice came over the intercom welcoming us and thanking us for choosing that airlines. He had a cheerful voice and told us that at the city we were flying into the weather was beautiful, sunny, and about 70 degrees. Suddenly, the plane roared to life and we were lifting off and headed through some thick, dark, and menacing clouds. Even that big jumbo jet rocked back and forth as it was buffeted by the clouds; but then all at once we broke through those dark and foreboding clouds and I looked out and the sun was shining everywhere, blue skies all around us. Those dark clouds were now behind us. I thought to myself, *If I could step out of that airplane I would walk on top of the clouds.* They were under my feet, behind me, and as I looked up and forward, all I could see was sun shiny blue skies. What was amazing was when I was entering the clouds beneath, they were dark, gray, and almost black looking, but when we broke through them and I looked down at them, they were white and looked like big fluffy pillows and I just wanted to jump out of that airplane and lay down on those big white clouds and rest.

What made the difference was the clouds were behind me and the sun was shining before me. It's kind of like traveling in your car down the highway and you look out through your windshield in front of you. You can see clearly in front of you and on each side of you and occasionally you will look into the rear view mirror. What would happen if you decided to look into your rear view mirror most of the time as you were driving down the highway? It wouldn't be long before you would find yourself off the road, in a ditch or in an accident. Well, it's the same way in life. If we are always looking back at the bad things that have happened in our lives, the regrets, the broken relationships, etc., it won't be long before we are discouraged and depressed. It's good to look back at the good times; and if you don't have even at least one good time in your past, then look back to learn from the past.

There is no way to escape stress in the world we live in today. It's all around us: where we work, where we vacation, where we eat, and, yes, even in our homes. The home, of all places, should be a sanctuary free from the kind of stress that affects us physiologically in a negative way. But way too often, as divorce rates indicate, the home is for many people where the majority of their stress comes from. But even in the sanctuary of your own home where you may be experiencing high levels of stress, there are solutions.

One of the ways I have dealt with stress ever since I had an understanding of what stress was (probably when I didn't get my way the first time as a child), I have always managed to have three plans available to me. I call them: Plan A, Plan B, and Plan C. I call it the ABC's of dealing with stress.

For instance, if you and your family have plans for a picnic on a particular day and the weather takes a turn for the worst, you need Plan B (some call it a backup plan) ready to implement, like going to the aquarium or going to the mall. Believe me, it will lower your stress if you have a Plan B or even further a Plan C when the kids start asking, "What are we going to do now, Mom?"

If I were to lock my keys in my truck today, I wouldn't become stressed at all because I keep another set along with my house keys in a magnet box hidden under my truck. That is my Plan B. Plan C is if for some reason that box has disappeared and I don't have an extra key—it's all good. Why? Because I know I made plans but I also realize even backup plans go awry sometimes—and that's okay. A lot of times we bring stress upon ourselves by how we run our lives.

Years ago, I knew a man who was a lineman for an electrical company in Kalamazoo, Michigan. I was about twenty-three years old and he was in his fifties. I was building a garage for him and one day he said to me, "Plan your work and work your plan." That sounds simple enough and it is, but it is so essential to reducing anxiety in your life. Now, some people live in a state of confusion without any plans and for the most part *appear* to be functioning just fine. *Appear* is the key word here. "Most men," Thoreau once wrote, "lead lives of quiet desperation."

Weimer Institute NEWSTART Lifestyle program is nestled in the Sierra foothills, forty-five minutes (forty miles) from Sacramento, California. It is a medical and educational institution treating and teaching people how to change their lifestyle so they can live happier and healthier lives.

They coined the acronym NEWSTART; but the principles have been around for millenniums. It is a simple concept of bringing eight natural laws of healing together to overcome diseases that we have either inherited or because of our choice of lifestyle we are living, we now have, or a combination of the two. Well, the Naked Truth is that through making simple changes in our lifestyle, we will experience significant changes, and we can either overcome these diseases or significantly reduce the symptoms we experience and finally reduce the amount of medication we are taking; and in most cases, get off the medications entirely.

I have taken their acronym and placed it across from the diseases that can be caused by a person's lifestyle that are listed in the column on the left. How many of the eight natural laws of healing that you incorporate into your lifestyle will determine how many lifestyle diseases you avoid, overcome, or at least reduce the symptoms you are already experiencing.

All eight natural laws of healing are listed in the column on the right that will help you overcome anyone or all of the lifestyle diseases (or at least reduce their symptoms) you see presented in the column on the left.

Diseases that lifestyle changes can effect	***Treatments:***
Lifestyle disease	NEWSTART
– Stress	Nutrition
– High blood pressure	Exercise
– Diabetes (adult onset)	Water
– **GERD** (Gastroesophageal reflux disease)	Sunshine
– Obesity	Temperance
– Depression	Air
– Cancer	Rest (sleep)
– AIDS	Trust in God

Taken from:
Total Life Ministries 3 TLM

On the chart above, look at the treatments on the right side; they are all things that don't cost a dime, but because pharmaceutical companies, hospitals, and doctors can't generate any money for these treatments, they are scorned as some type of voodoo or something to stay away from.

I would like to look at each of the natural laws of healing listed under the acronym NEWSTART:

Nutrition

Change to a plant-based diet of wholesome grains, nuts, fruits, and vegetables.

Eat more sparingly.

Leave the dinner table a little hungry; this will keep you from overeating.

Thirty minutes to an hour before eating, drink a glass or two of water; this will give you a feeling of fullness and you will eat less.

Chew your food thoroughly; this will keep your stomach from working so hard and from secreting so much acid to break up the undigested food.

Eat slowly. It takes about twenty minutes for your stomach to send a signal to your brain that you are full.

Drink at least two glasses of water between meals.

Don't drink with your meals; but if you do, don't drink ice cold drinks. Ice cold drinks impede digestion. The ice cold drink chills your stomach and small intestine and your body now has to warm those organs up before real digestion begins.

There are basically 4 reasons you drink with your meals.

1. The food is too spicy hot
2. You don't chew your food thoroughly enough. If you observe people in fast food restaurants, they will take a bike of burger and fries and then wash that food down with a soda pop.
3. You're not drinking enough water between meals.
4. It is a habit of our lifestyle to have a drink of something with our meals.

Have a minimum of three hours between meals. Four hours are better and five hours between meals is best. This applies to the time between your last meal of the day and the time you go to bed.

Exercise

There are three forms of exercise that you need at least three days a week—more is preferable.

1. Cardiovascular
   Walking
   Swimming
   Running
   Biking
   Racquet ball
   Gardening

I've just listed a few; but whatever you do for cardiovascular, make it last for at least twenty minutes.

Some people ask me, "How fast should I run?" My answer is, "If you can't carry on a conversation with someone, you're running too fast.

Don't exercise in excess, because if you do, you'll end up burning muscle instead of fat. Muscle is the largest fat burning organ you have and that is why you need strength training as part of your exercise program.

2. Strength training
   Weight lifting
   Push-ups
   Chin ups-pull ups
   Isometric

3. Stretching
   This is one area that is often missed in an exercise program—but it is extremely important.
   As with any exercise, don't forget about proper breathing, especially deep breathing-slowly.

And whatever you do for exercise, do with a cheerful heart and you'll begin to lower your stress. Some people say, "I'm going to exercise if it kills me," and it may if you approach exercise with a negative attitude.

You'll hear now and again how someone suddenly died who was a faithful runner and he exercised almost every day. You might be thinking, *I thought exercise would make you live longer*. It will; but exercise doesn't really remove plaque from your arteries—only diet will do that.

Water

The human body is made up of about 75 percent water, therefore our bodies need water every day.

If you drink two glasses of water when you first get up in the morning, then between breakfast and lunch, drink another two glasses of water, then another two glasses after lunch but before supper, and finally two glasses after supper; you will have drank eight glasses of water. Increase this amount if you're exercising or working outside in the heat.

Can you actually drink too much water? I guess you can, but consuming too much water is not a problem for most people.

Drinking coffee, tea, or soda pops does not count as drinking water. Coffee, tea, and soda pops actually dehydrate our bodies, thus making us more thirsty for water; so when you are thirsty, drink water—it's the only drink that will truly quench our thirst. Coffee, tea, and soda pops and alcohol are manufactured to keep you coming back for more of the same. These drinks don't encourage you to drink more water.

You'll save a lot of money by just drinking water, so long as you don't buy into the idea that you can only drink bottled water. Most bottled water comes from the same treatment processing plant that comes into your homes. Some call that water-"from the toilet to the tap".

In our home, we have a small filter system that I paid about $100.00 for at Lowe's. The water tastes great and it's a good idea once in a while to have your water tested that you use for drinking.

Drinking water lowers your blood pressure and your cholesterol and thins your blood so you are at a lower risk for a heart attack and stroke. Your mind will become clearer and sharper, especially if you have quit drinking soda pop, coffee and alcohol.

Sunshine

We all need sunshine—every day if possible; but it only takes about fifteen minutes of just simply standing outside waiting for a bus, working in the garden, taking a walk, or talking with neighbors to get all the sun we need.

I know that many people use tanning beds on a regular basis and some people use tanning beds when they expect to go to the beach for a vacation. I don't recommend the use of tanning beds at all. If you want to lie out, then do it in fifteen-twenty-thirty-forty-five-minute increments. Work your way up in time and avoid the use of sun tan lotions. You won't need them if you limit your exposure time, and you'll get a beautiful tan.

Wherever you live, make sure you get plenty of sunlight in your home. Don't have trees up close to your house. Open up the drapes or curtains in the morning and let the fresh beautiful sunlight stream into your home.

Sunshine will kill germs that are on our furniture and counters. After you first get up, don't make your bed right away; wait until after breakfast or wait until the sunlight has had an opportunity to kill the germs in your beds.

Notice what cats and dogs do during the day: They search out a place where they can soak up some sun rays. Sunshine lowers our stress levels and strengthens our immune systems.

Temperance

I have had people ask me if I believe in moderation in all things. My answer is a resounding no.

In everything that is good, do it in moderation. In everything that is bad, abstain from it.

If you do this, you'll be temperate in all things.

Air

Wow! How important is air? Try going without it for a few minutes. Actually, I don't recommend you to go without air because we all would cease to exist within a few minutes without air to breathe.

Every morning after you get up and before you drink your two glasses of water, do some deep breathing exercises; it will only take a few minutes. We all need to learn how to breathe deeply. This is one of the reasons throughout the day we are tired especially those who have sedentary lifestyles or who sit at desks all day. Our blood becomes sluggish because there isn't enough fresh oxygen available and carbon dioxide is building up in the body. Practice deep breathing throughout the day and you will notice you have more energy and you are less likely to get sleepy. Proper breathing will help your complexion, your attitude, your productivity in the work place, your concentration, your meditation, your interpersonal relationships just to name a few.

At our home, we keep our windows opened just enough to let in fresh air. If your windows are closed and there is no fresh supply of free flowing air, you are breathing only positive ions; we also need negative ions and that's what we get when we let fresh air into our homes every day.

Rest

Adults need between seven and nine hours of sleep each night. Later in the book, I talk about getting two or three hours of your sleep before midnight, because that's the time that the stress-lowering hormones are secreted. Don't let the television or the computer rob you of your sleep.

Try to be consistent in your sleep patterns even on the weekends. People who eat late at night will toss and turn more and will not be as refreshed in the morning when they arise.

If you're on sleeping pills or some other kind of sleep aides, get off them as soon as you are able to. These drugs will rob you of true sleep. If you keep taking something to help you sleep, you eventually need something stronger and this is where the danger lies.

Trust in God

I would be remiss if I didn't put God into the equation when making lifestyle changes. You can eat all the right things, exercise every day, get plenty of rest, drink plenty of water, never drink alcohol, never smoke, never take drugs and still end up dying of cancer.

Once I heard of a woman who had a terminal disease and sought the traditional avenue of medication/drugs and surgery. After spending all that she had on medical and doctor bills, she finally reached out to God. She had trusted in her doctor and the hospital to guide her to health but never knew or considered where true healing comes from. Doctors and hospitals can't heal anyone—only God can heal.

A few years ago, my wife and I were traveling on Interstate 4 going through Orlando, Florida, when we noticed on the city buses a slogan that read, "Florida Hospital, making miracles through magic."

I asked my wife, "Isn't that the Florida Hospital that is owned by the Seventh-Day-Adventist Church?"

"Of course," she responded, "yes."

Somehow, Florida Hospital had some connection with Disney World and somebody in the Public Relations department thought this would be a cute advertisement; or it was Disney World's idea; but somehow, it found its way onto the city buses of Orlando.

In any case, it takes away the origin where true healing really comes from. There is no magic in true healing of the body and the mind. There is no waving a wand over someone and presto, one is healed. Many people are not healed from diseases they have because most people don't want to change their lifestyles.

Just the other day, I was leaving my apartment and as I walked down the stairs, I encountered two other people. The lady looked to be in her seventies and the man probably in his forties. It looked like he was assisting her to wherever she was going. He said to me, "Hampton, you need to pray for this lady because she has blockages in the arteries of her legs and in her neck—she's just not feeling good.

Then it suddenly dawned upon me this was the same lady who was up early in the morning smoking, the smoke always wafting up to my apartment that I have to shut the door. When he asked me to pray for her, I knew he meant for healing. But would she change her lifestyle if God chose to heal her? Probably not. The reason she had the blocked arteries was because of her smoking and other negative lifestyle choices she had made.

I kindly responded, "I'll pray that she can quit smoking," and then I explained that smoking was, at least, one of the contributing factors of her present condition.

When I was a little boy, even before I first went to school, it was my job to tend to our flock of about thirty-five goats. On occasion, one of our male family members would also be with me in the fields helping me take care of the goats.

My mother made goat cheese and we sold the goat cheese and the goats' milk in our health food store in town in the city of Hot Springs, Arkansas.

One day, this person and I had a break after the goats had been tended to and he made me perform oral sex on him while he sat on a log in the middle of the field. He threatened me that if I didn't, he would hurt me. No one else was around; I had no one to call upon for help. Part of the reason I didn't tell anyone, especially my parents, wasn't just because he threatened me, but because I was too embarrassed and I felt too ashamed.

Well, last year that person was coming to visit my family with his wife. I hadn't seen him for twenty years. Knowing he was coming, I felt I needed to bring closure to that incident and help him do the same. They were at our house for the weekend and I had to travel out of town before they left. I kept thinking I need to say something to him. On Monday morning, after saying bye to my wife, he followed me out the door to my truck. I opened my door and turned around and looked him straight in the eyes and said, "I want you to know that I forgive you for molesting me when I was a little boy" and I specifically stated what he'd done.

He seemed surprised and responded, "I don't remember, I'm sorry."

The only reason I share this story is because too many people today are living with hurt, shame, embarrassment, and resentment over things that were said or done to them at some time in their lives.

The Penn State scandal has taken first place in the news. "Jerry Sandusky, retired Penn State defensive Coordinator, is charged with having sexually abused 8 boys over 15 years and has maintained his innocence."

Mike McQueary, "told the grand jury he was distraught by what he witnessed and walked away after both Sandusky and the boy saw him."

Penn State head coach Joe Paterno was fired and he is now seeking a lawyer. Jerry Sandusky after being arrested and booked is now out walking the streets on a hundred thousand dollar bail.

Is there something wrong with this picture? Coach Mike McQueary who witnessed Sandusky molesting this boy in the shower walked away after the boy saw him and then "met the minimum" "obligation of reporting what he saw to his superiors who are required under Pennsylvania law to report such assaults to authorities."

Why didn't you, Mike McQueary, go into that shower and rescue that boy? What were you afraid of Mike? You need to take a good look at yourself, because that boy that was being viciously attacked by Jerry Sandusky got a good look at you.

Where are the noble men and women of this generation who will dare risk their relationships, their reputations, their jobs, their marriages, yes, and even their lives to intervene to save a little boy or girl from sexual molestation.

What-was there a virus in the air that Jerry Sandusky caught that made him molest these boys? I hear people say, "he's sick". Let me tell you, he may be sick because of the demons that possess him now; but he wasn't sick years ago when he made a conscious decision to begin formulating in his mind what he eventually followed through with.

Go with me into the mind of that boy Jerry Sandusky was viciously raping in the shower; now look through his eyes as his eyes meet Mike McQueary's eyes and for just a moment, he's thinking, this guy will stop this man from raping me, but then he sees him leave and Jerry Sandusky continues his vicious, reprehensible, disgraceful, disgusting, immoral, and absolutely sickening molestation.

Judge Jenine has a program on the Fox network and after discussing the Penn State incident with other Lawyers, she wrapped up her segment with this statement: "There is a special place in hell reserved for you who molest children."

For me that incident affected my relationship with both sexes; but I didn't understand that for years. I'm sure this will be true of these boys that Jerry Sandusky molested. If any of you boys, now young men probably, are reading this book—I want you to know there is hope. I made it out of the jungle of shame, pain and hurt. One day I dared look back into the past and I faced it, I addressed it and I moved forward. I decided I wasn't going to let the past steal my joy. I was convinced for years it was my fault these things happened to me, but I know now it wasn't my fault and I can assure you, my friends, it was not your fault either.

Resentment can and will destroy you if you don't face it; deal with it and move on. I do believe there are times you may need the professional services of a good Christian counselor, such as a psychologist or psychiatrist.

If you do need to have counseling, don't let it drag on and on and keep bringing up the past anew.

But be very careful who you send your children to for counseling. I was 16 years of age and I was having some adjustment problems and a judge ordered that I see a psychiatrist. I don't know who made the decision as to who the psychiatrist was I would see, but after only a few sessions, he proceeded to touch me inappropriately and I made the decision never to return to him and all agreed.

As with most areas of medicine, psychiatrists many times just put their patients on some type of drug and move on to the next patient on the schedule. Again, the best treatment and advice coming from a counselor should first be about making changes in your lifestyle that will help you cope with issues you may be struggling with.

Jennifer Gardner Trulson has written a book, *Where You Left Me*, and just recently she was interviewed about losing her husband during 911. She is an attorney and now an author and remarried. At the end of that interview, she said, "You don't have to close the door to live in the present, you can carry the lost with you."

In recent years, research has pointed to the positive effects that religiosity, faith, spirituality, prayer, forgiveness, hope, and church attendance can have on health, including mental health.

Numerous prominent scientific publications have reported a connection between religious faith and positive mental and emotional well-being. Surprise of surprises! Not really.

Yet, this is no magic; the faith factor applies only to those who are deeply committed to their religious principles. Psychiatrist Montagu Barker, an expert in the interface between religion and mental health, states that "Religion is a potent safeguard against mental illness, but only when believers possess a strong commitment to their beliefs. If not, religion may become a source of guilt and the cause of emotional, mental, and behavioral disturbances."

In a truly Christian home where love rules supreme, it will be a place where we give our own the best, where the simple attentions and courtesies of courtship come as naturally as the day they were born.

I found the following story tucked away in a little book entitled *I Met a Miracle* written by George E. Vandeman who started the religious television program, *It Is Written*.

Some years ago, a couple were about to celebrate their golden wedding anniversary, and a local newspaper sent out a reporter for an interview and found the husband was at home.

"What is your recipe for a long, happy marriage?" the reporter asked.

"Well, I'll tell you, young fellow," the old gentleman said slowly. "I was an orphan, and I always had to work pretty hard for my board and keep. I never even looked at a girl until I was grown. Sarah was the first one I ever kept company with. When she *maneuvered me into proposing*, I was scared stiff, but after the wedding, her pa took me aside and handed me a little package. 'Here is all you really need to know,' he said. And this is it." He reached for a large gold watch in his pocket, opened it, and handed it to the reporter. There across the face of the watch, where he could see it a dozen times a day, were written these words: "Say something nice to Sarah."

He goes on to write in his book about the above story:

> Too simple to work? Just remember that great happiness is made up of little kindnesses. It is also true that a lack of appreciation in small things may grow until it becomes a great divisive factor.

> The ruin of a marriage may not be a dramatic affair. There may be no unfaithfulness, no desertion, no blows—just a slow accumulation of dissatisfaction, a gradual growth of misunderstandings and irritations, until one day one companion or the other says, "I can't stand it any longer." And the tragedy is that many such individuals do not really sense what is happening or how to stop it.
>
> Remember this: Unsolved problems become set in the mind as attitudes. Try making it a rule never to go to sleep at night until disagreements are settled.
>
> I believe the most powerful words ever spoken in this world, at least next to, "I was wrong" or "I forgive you," are "I love you."

Many people will admit they were wrong because they don't want to lose their job or their marriage; but it takes love—real love to say "I was wrong" for no other reason than that you have hurt someone.

New York Congressman Weiner over this last weekend said to reporters that he didn't send that "bulging underwear" text to that woman. He denied the allegations to every reporter (at least that was a bipartisan move) over and over again for more than a week; but then yesterday, he came out and admitted to it and added that over three years, he had corresponded with a total of six women in the same manner. Why would he lie at first and then just a few days later admit that he had lied? He said he lied because he wanted to protect his wife and family and that he was just ashamed. I'll give him that; but I might add he also did so because this is an election year and he doesn't want to lose his job and the whole democratic machinery doesn't want his vacant Senate seat to go to the GOP. Also, Congressman Weiner had his eyes on becoming mayor of New York City in 2013. I believe this because he emphatically stated, "I'm not resigning." His not resigning seems more important to him than the hurt he has brought to his family, friends and political supporters.

Why should anyone believe anything Congressman Weiner says after emphatically lying to reporters for an entire week? Barbara Walters was reported as saying, "Maybe he was just trying to sext his wife and his sext message got intercepted." Congressman Weiner admitted sexting six women over a three-year period. Could all of those been sent to his wife? No, the sad fact remains, he and many others in Washington like him just got caught and they are truly sorry for that; they are not sorry for their immorality. It is reprehensible for any leader to be involved in immoral activity especially as a congressman.

This is clearly another reason we have so many people on so many mind-altering drugs; very few people really want to take responsibility for their own actions. If people were to step up to the plate and assume responsibility for their own actions, we wouldn't need so many psychiatrists and psychologists.

If you have had something happen in your childhood or when you were growing up that devastated you, you need to travel back in time and settle this incident or incidents if it is in your power to do so.

A few years back, we had the principal of our high school abruptly fired. Why? A woman came forward and stated years ago when she was a little girl, this man had molested her. He admitted to that charge and was immediately fired.

This is one way you may have to deal with something like this. But once you have gone back and have dealt with whatever it is that happened in your life, then move on and begin to soar with the eagles on wings of thanksgiving; because when you do this, you'll feel a great relief and freedom. Don't stay around in the psychiatrist's or psychologist's chair week after week talking the same things over; that's what I call pecking with chickens.

If you have cut yourself and a scab develops and you keep picking at the scab, it may never heal. How many times have I heard mothers tell their little ones when she would see them picking at a scab on their leg, "That's never going to heal if you keep picking at it." The same applies when you keep rehearsing what has happened to you. You must bring closure to those old psychological and maybe physical scars; if you don't, you cannot interact at 100 percent with other family members and friends. That's the Naked Truth.

Congressman Weiner also stated that he really loves his wife and that she loves him and they are not going to break-up over the bulging underwear incidents.

Now if Senator Weiner has said, "I'm sorry—I have done wrong" out of love, his stress level will really go down; but if he is saying it to only save face, his immune system will be affected negatively because of the increase stress he will experience.

When unfaithfulness occurs as in the cases of former President Clinton, Mark Foley, John Edwards, and now Anthony Weiner, physiological changes take place in the lives of the innocent and or the guilty.

Bill Clinton had and continues to have heart issues. When you are unfaithful, you are bringing upon yourself untold stress. I heard years ago of a study that was done about the impact of sex on the heart. What was interesting in the study was that sex did not hurt the heart unless you were having sex with someone other than your wife.

But, in cases like John Edwards, his wife Elizabeth dies after struggling with cancer. You might be thinking, "but didn't she have cancer before John had his affair and had a child out of wedlock." Maybe, but if John Edwards had been faithful to her, she may have overcome her cancer; but maybe she wouldn't have—we'll never know now.

No one will ever know what kind of stress men and women go through when their spouses are unfaithful.

I've heard reported that Anthony Weiner's wife is pregnant. The stress that his wife is dealing with right now over the news of his unfaithfulness is having and will continue to have a negative effect on the unborn child. Congressman Weiner's porn addiction will be passed down to his children and then to their children if someone doesn't say, "Enough!" and tries to change their lifestyle.

Men, when you have an affair on your wife, the ripple effect to family and friends never ends. You are telling the world, "I don't love this woman" and you are basically throwing her under the bus. You're telling your kids that sex with another woman and instant gratification is more important than my love for you. I have chosen sex with lust over my love for you.

One of the greatest reasons America is in the moral decay it is in is the fabric of the family has been fractured.

ADHD, for the most part, could be resolved if the home became a safe haven, radiating with love and security where children heard their parents tell each other "I love you."

Also, if children were given the opportunity to just be children at home spending time with their mom or dad, ADHD wouldn't have a chance of surviving. But when children come from broken homes where they have heard their parents yelling at each other, they sometimes become nervous wrecks; and instead of the parents making changes and concessions in their lives, they seek out a doctor or psychiatrist who will put little Johnny or little Susie on some form of poisonous drug, just because they don't want to deal with the situation.

In many cases, the sickness of children can be traced to errors in management. Irregularities in eating, insufficient clothing in the chilly evening, lack of vigorous exercise to keep the blood in healthy circulation, or lack of abundance of air for its purification, may be the cause of the trouble. Let the parents study to find the causes of the sickness and then remedy the wrong conditions as soon as possible.

Children are generally brought up from the cradle to indulge the appetite and are taught that they live to eat. The mother does much toward the formation of the character of her children in their childhood. She can teach them to control the appetite, or she can teach them to indulge the appetite and become gluttons. The mother often arranges her plans to accomplish a certain amount through the day; and when the children trouble her, instead of taking time to soothe their little sorrows and divert them, something is given them to eat to keep them still, which answers the purpose for a short time but eventually makes things worse. The children's stomachs have been pressed with food, when they had not the least want of it. All that was required was a little of the mother's time and attention. But she regarded her time as altogether too precious to devote to the amusement of her children. Perhaps the arrangement of her house in a tasteful manner for visitors to praise, and to have her food cooked in a fashionable style are with her higher considerations than the happiness and health of her children.

And please, mothers and fathers, I implore you when you're out with your children to have fun don't let the cell phone distract you from spending time with your children. At the park where my wife and I take our little girls to play, so often we see parents either texting or playing games on their cell phones and sometimes they are clueless to what's happening with their children. Don't make that mistake.

Someday, parents will have to deal with a son or daughter who has been on drugs to treat ADHD and it is usually not a pretty picture. You will someday have to deal with the situation.

Before leaving this chapter on stress, I want to share with you *36 Christian Ways to Reduce Stress*. I used this when I taught lifestyle change classes at Eden Valley located in Colorado not far from Estes Park. Eden Valley is mentioned in the back of this book as one of the lifestyle centers I recommend if you are seeking help to live healthier and happier lives.

1. Pray
2 Go to bed on time.
3 Get up on time so you can start the day unrushed.
4 Say "No," to projects/activities that won't fit into your time schedule, or that will compromise your mental health.
5 Delegate tasks to capable others.
6 Simplify and unclutter your life.
7 Less is more (Although one is often not enough, two are often too many.).
8 Allow extra time to do things and to get to places.
9 Pace yourself. Spread out big changes and difficult projects over time; don't lump the hard things all together.
10 Take one day at a time.
11 Separate worries from concerns. If a situation is a concern, find out what God would have you to do and let go of the anxiety. If you can't do anything about a situation, forget it.
12 Live within your budget.

13 Have backups; an extra car key in your wallet, an extra house key buried in the garden, extra stamps, etc.
14 K. M. S. (Keep Mouth Shut.) This single piece of advice can prevent an enormous amount of trouble.
15 Do something for the kid in ***you*** every day.
16 Carry a Bible with you to read while waiting in line.
17 Get enough exercise.
18 Eat right.
19 Get organized so everything has its place.
20 While driving, listen to a tape that can help improve your quality of life.
21 Write thoughts and inspirations down.
22 Every day, find time to be alone.
23 Having problems? Talk to God on the spot. Try to nip small problems in the bud. Don't wait until it's time to go to bed to try and pray.
24 Make friends with Godly people.
25 Keep a folder of favorite scriptures on hand.
26 Remember that the shortest bridge between despair and hope is often a good "Thank you, Jesus!"
27 Laugh.
28 Laugh some more!
29 Take your work seriously, but yourself not at all.
30 Develop a forgiving attitude (Most people are doing the best they can).
31 Be kind to unkind people (They probably need it the most).
32 Sit on your ego.
33 Talk less; listen more.
34 Slow down.
35 Remind yourself that you are not the general manager of the universe.
36 Every night before bed, think of one thing you're grateful for that you've never been grateful for before.

The reason I put so much stress on stress is because this is the origin of many ailments and diseases, both physical and especially mental. If you can learn how to deal with stress, you can accomplish anything.

Fear is where a lot of our stresses come from. Don't let the stress of fear rob you of your joy.

Chapter Five: High Blood Pressure (HTN Hypertension)

How Is Your Blood Pressure Measured?

Right on the front end of this chapter I want to say the quickest way to lower your blood pressure is to eat a plant-based diet or a diet high in fruits and vegetables. If you just cut out red meats your blood pressure will come down; but if you want to be in optimum health, then cut out all meat, including fish and chicken. Not only will your blood pressure come down, but so will your weight.

Blood pressure is expressed as two numbers. These numbers represent the pressure against the walls of your blood vessels as the blood moves through them. Systolic pressure is when pressure is highest in the arteries and occurs when the heart contracts. Diastolic pressure is the moment of minimum pressure in the arteries and occurs when the heart relaxes. Normal blood pressure is less than 120 (systolic) over 80 (diastolic), typically written as 120/80 mm Hg (read 120 over 80 millimeters of mercury).1

What the Numbers Mean:

If your blood pressure is less than 120/80, your blood pressure is normal.

If your blood pressure is between 120/80 and 140/90, you're at risk for high blood pressure. Lifestyle modifications are important and should be recommended by your doctor or healthcare professional if your blood pressure is 140/90 and above or 130/80 and above and you have diabetes or chronic kidney disease, or your blood pressure is high. Lifestyle modifications and high blood pressure medications are important and should be recommended by your doctor or healthcare professionals.

If you're making lifestyle changes and your doctor has started you on blood pressure lowering medications, he will see a drastic change in your blood pressure within thirty days and should recommend cutting back and finally getting off entirely of the blood pressure medications.

Causes and Symptoms of High Blood Pressure:

What causes high blood pressure?

For 85 percent to 95 percent of people with high blood pressure, the cause of their high blood pressure is not known. Called primary hypertension, this condition probably results from a variety of causes.

Risk factors:

1. Age and Sex. The risk of developing high blood pressure increases as you age. Most cases of high blood pressure are diagnosed in men until the age of forty-five. From age forty-five to fifty-four, men and women are equally at risk for high blood pressure. After the age of fifty-four, women are actually more likely to have high blood pressure than men. This may suggest that estrogen has a protective role in blood pressure. It is thought that estrogen helps keep blood vessels flexible. Estrogen may also work with other hormones to reduce the risk of high blood pressure in younger women.
2. Family History. People with relatives who have high blood pressure are more likely to develop high blood pressure; the key is "are likely to develop high blood pressure," because by making some simple lifestyle changes, you will not suffer with high blood pressure like other members of your family.
3. Ethnicity. People of African American and Native American ethnicity have very high rates of high blood pressure,

and the situation appears to be a growing problem. Compared with Caucasians, African Americans develop hypertension earlier in life, and their average blood pressures are much higher.

4. Diet. People who regularly eat foods that are high in salt are more susceptible to high blood pressure. This is really true of processed foods and of eating out. Avoid both as much as possible.

5. Obesity. People who are overweight are at risk for many illnesses, including high blood pressure.

6. Stress. Studies have shown that people with heightened anxiety, intense anger, and suppressed expression of anger were more at risk of developing high blood pressure. This is your typical type "A" personality. I would love to walk into Wall Street on a busy Monday morning and get blood pressure readings on all the Wall Street brokers.

Some complications of hypertension or high blood pressure are:

- stroke
- congestive heart failure
- heart attack
- atherosclerosis (hardening of the arteries)
- aneurysm
- kidney disease
- disease of the retina
- blood vessel rupture
- weakened memory and mental ability
- decreased libido

This isn't a complete list; but it's a start. From looking at this list, one can tell why high blood pressure is called the "silent killer"? This is really played out for the person who has had an aneurysm since birth. I remember an administrator who came home after work and sometime in the evening he said to his wife, "My head hurts," and he laid back on his bed with his wife by his side and died right there on the spot from a ruptured cerebral aneurysm. They performed an autopsy and discovered he had a congenital cerebral aneurysm. He never was aware that he was born with a cerebral aneurysm. Maybe if he had not had high blood pressure, the aneurysm would not have ruptured; but I can tell you this: Uncontrolled high blood pressure does raise the risk factor a few notches.

"Control of blood pressure begins with knowing what your blood pressure is. Do not assume that just because you feel fine you are free of blood pressure problems. High blood pressure is indeed called "the silent killer." It has this name because serious disability or death is often the very first symptom of hypertension. Many people will never realize that their blood pressure is high unless they get it checked by a doctor, go to a screening program, or get a blood pressure instrument and check it themselves. In fact, it is common for people to feel fine with blood pressures of 200/100 or even higher. Indeed, you may feel great while being unwittingly on the verge of a disaster such as a sudden stroke or heart attack, or gradual kidney damage with resulting renal failure down the road," (*Proof Positive*, Neil Nedley, M.D. pg. 130).

If you are one of those who take medication to control your high blood pressure, you will eventually have complications from the effects of the medications you are ingesting. Every medication you take has an effect on your body in some negative way. This is why many people find themselves on other medications to try to control the negative effects of the first drug prescribed for them. It is a viscous cycle that can and will have a negative effect in the long run, because most of the effects of these drugs go unnoticed. Also, the cost of medications is very expensive. It is always better to lower your blood pressure through making simple lifestyle changes. The naked truth is medications change the way you think, the way you react to certain situations, and the way you see life.

We often tell our children all the bad effects of drugs and how these drugs can change them permanently and cut their lives short, yet all the while having a medicine cabinet chucked full of drug medications.

Many people can't get up in the morning without a drug like caffeine; they have to have drugs like caffeine all throughout the day, and they can't go to sleep without a drug. What does that sound like to you? I think addiction would sum up that whole scenario.

If you don't want your kids on drugs, and I'm sure you don't, then limit medication to only what you must take; and guess what, you will feel better, you will look better, and you will have more money in your pocket and your kids will be less likely to take drugs.

Nearly seventy-five million Americans have a potentially life-threatening disease—and twenty-eight percent don't even know it. According to a new study from the National Heart, Lung, and Blood Institute (NHLBI), more adults than ever in the U.S. have high blood pressure. In fact, this is the scariest part: Because it doesn't usually cause symptoms, by the time some people realize they have high blood pressure (a.k.a. hypertension), it already may have caused significant damage in the form of heart disease, stroke, vision or kidney problems, or, in men, erectile dysfunction.

Research shows conclusively that the most common day for heart attacks is Monday. Statistics spike on Monday mornings, in particular, since heart attacks occur between 4:00 A.M. and 10:00 A.M. more than any other six-hour period. The Women's Heart Foundation notes that blood platelets are stickier in the morning hours, which can contribute to an attack; this is another reason you want to make sure you are drinking plenty of fresh cool water. How much water should you drink a day? Just follow this guideline and you'll never go wrong. When you first get up in the morning, drink two eight-ounce glasses of water preferably about an hour before that big breakfast you're going to eat. Mid-morning and at least two hours after you have finished breakfast drink two eight-ounce glasses of water. Again, about two hours after lunch, drink another two eight-ounce glasses of water; and, finally, about two hours after dinner, drink your final two glasses of water. This schedule of drinking water will give you eight glasses of water a day. This should be the minimum amount each day.

Drinking water will lower your cholesterol and decrease the viscosity of your blood, both of which will help prevent a heart attack and stroke.

Every day, I take a history from patients who are going to have surgery or are having a procedure done like a colonoscopy. A great number of these patients are on antihypertensive medications. They are not always taking them for blood pressure issues; sometimes they have been prescribed by their doctor to slow the heart or to reduce a tremor in their hands. But whatever the reason the patient is taking these medications, they are definitely affecting other organs in their bodies even if they don't have high blood pressure.

Any medication or drug you are taking does have an effect on the body and the brain. For some people, they may have to be on some particular drug for the rest of their lives; but this happens to be the minority.

If you are one of those who are taking a medication for the rest of your life, don't be discouraged or disheartened. When you begin making lifestyle changes, the amount of medication you're taking may be reduced. Always consult your physician before cutting back on the amount of medication you're taking. If a doctor refuses to work with you in adjusting your treatment, then shop around for a physician who believes in making lifestyle changes a component of good health. More physicians are realizing how important lifestyle changes are in treating patients. Look for a physician who believes in preventing diseases by changing your lifestyle.

At the end of this book, I have a list of Lifestyle Centers that you may contact to either join one of their programs or get some advice and answers over the phone.

Preventive healthcare should be affordable to everyone, everywhere all across this great country.

When President Obama first began working on healthcare reform, I listened as he said, "If we can get people off some of these medications or drugs, and institute some basic lifestyle changes, we can save a lot of money." He was right. I have not heard him mention another statement like that. Why? Well, the biggest roadblock to preventive medicine (making simple lifestyle changes) is the trillion-dollar pharmaceutical companies or the legal drug cartels. If they cannot make money on giving you good health, they don't want to hear what you have to say. Actually, they don't want you to have good health because they would be out of business. I say again, "Drugs don't cure."

Let me put this as succinctly and clearly as I know how: Healing comes from God, physicians treat symptoms. Physicians cannot heal you—only God can heal.

Last weekend, I had dinner with an elderly couple who this year will both turn eighty-one. They are both in good health, of a sound mind, and physically very active. They are Seventh-Day-Adventists residing in a small town in Tennessee. The husband's mother lived until she was ninety-six and the wife's mother lived until she was ninety-seven. They definitely have longevity in their families; but they also follow good lifestyle principles. The wife told me a story of a woman she knew recently who was dying and she visited her at the hospital. The patient was on a long list of medications. She commented to my friend who was visiting her, "With all these medications I'm taking you would think I should be the healthiest person in the world." Three days later, she died.

I will say that the more medications you're taking, the more unhealthy you are. The two are inversely related. As you take more medications, your health goes down; as you take less medications, you have better health.

Every medication you take affects the body and mind and the more you take, the greater the effect for harm, not good.

If a drug could cure high blood pressure, then at some point, you could stop taking the drug and presto, like magic, you are cured. But, that is not the case. If you suddenly stop taking high blood pressure medication, you may experience a rebound affect. Your blood pressure may rebound to a dangerously high level. So even when you begin making some simple lifestyle changes, you need to taper off your medication over a month or so. This is why the drug companies tell you to consult your doctor before stopping a medication. They know these drugs can kill you. If you stop taking them suddenly and you die, they have lost an investment—you. If you continue taking them, you'll still die but only after they have sucked you dry financially. They don't care. If they truly cared about your health, and you needed to be on a medication, they would make these drugs affordable to everyone everywhere.

My mother, a registered nurse for over fifty years, and graduate of Hinsdale Hospital, a diploma program, once said, "If you give antibiotics, you will get well in a week, but if you don't take antibiotics, you will be well in seven days." She was really referring to the common colds that we all suffer from. We now know that antibiotics really don't help in treating a common cold, except, in the care of a secondary infection. But back in the forties after WWII when antibiotics were introduced, they were given out like candy for everything and to everyone. And now, as a result of overuse of antibiotics, there has developed resistant strains of microorganisms that most antibiotics won't touch. So scientists and pharmaceutical companies are scrambling to come up with the next generation of powerful antibiotics to kill the new resistant strains of germs.

I have said earlier that the single most important thing you can do for yourself and your family financially is to start making simple lifestyle changes. There is also another important reason to make these changes. These medications or drugs may not always be available as they are now. An easy way to do away with a large elderly population is just not make the drugs accessible. When a government is having a financial crises like our country is having, the sanctity of life isn't always at the top of their priority list. Both extremes of life (the unborn and the elderly) are in danger.

The good news is you can take control of your life once again, and for the most part, it will not cost you a dime. No, you don't need to buy a membership down at the local health club. I'm not saying health clubs are bad. They're not. Sometimes you get encouragement from trainers and other people you meet that attend the health club on a regular schedule. But, if at first you don't have the money to shell out for a membership at a local club, or you don't have the time, then do your work out at home.

Here is some interesting information on health clubs and home gym equipment. Gym memberships are a nineteen-billion-dollar-a-year business. Eighty percent of memberships are not used. Memberships last about three weeks. Well, you might be thinking, *I'll just invest in some home gym equipment.* Home exercise equipment is a four-billion-dollar-a-year business. Eighty percent of the equipment is not used after about three weeks. Well, what about diets? Diets lasts about seventy-two hours, so they are your single worst investment in seeking good health; and, remember when you remove the letter "T" from diet, you are left with the word "die".

I live in Tennessee at the present time but we still own a home in Colorado. All my weights and work out equipment are in Colorado at our other home. When I go back to close on the house, I'll pick up my equipment. For now, though, I went to Dick's Sports and purchased a chin up bar and pushup handles. It also came with a DVD. It shows you how to have a thirty-minute workout each day in your own home. It only cost $59.00.

I recommend that everyone do strength training on a regular schedule. As we grow older, we lose muscle; and muscle is the largest fat burning organ in the body. And this fact becomes very important when we come to the chapter on obesity.

When you work out for strength training and if you are lifting weights, limit your work out to 45 minutes. Within the first 45 minutes testosterone and growth hormones increase and you need this to build muscle; but after 45 minutes the hormone cortisol increases and begins to break down your muscles and since muscle is the largest fat burning organ in the body, you will now actually start putting on weight through fat gain.

Salt is a major culprit in causing high blood pressure. If you eat out a lot, especially at fast food restaurants, you're getting way too much salt. Most foods you buy at grocery stores are loaded with salt, especially crackers, chips, and many other finger foods.

"Salt consists of two elements—sodium and chloride; it is forty percent sodium. It is found in a majority of foods in the supermarket, and the amount per serving is listed (as sodium) on the container or package by law. Surprisingly, research suggests that it is actually the combination of sodium with chloride that does the damage. In animal studies on high blood pressure, neither excess sodium alone nor excess chloride alone causes high blood pressure. However, the labeling of sodium content usually provides the necessary information: sodium and chloride typically are found in roughly equal amounts in foods. Thus, by limiting the sodium intake, we generally limit the chloride intake as well," (*Proof Positive*, Neil Nedley, M.D. pg 137).

If you want to lower your blood pressure without taking medications, then institute some simple lifestyle changes, like:

If you're a meat eater, change to a plant based diet—become a vegetarian. If you still choose to eat meat, then cut out or cut back on red meat consumption. Eat more fresh fruits, vegetables and grains, and eat an ounce of nuts a day—unsalted. Try walnuts, almonds, or pecans. I eat an ounce of pecans or walnuts almost every day for my protein intake and that takes away my desire for more protein and for my desire for eggs every day.

If you're going to eat eggs, make sure you buy the ones that have written on the outside of the carton, "open or free range and no antibiotics, steroids, or growth hormones, but fed only with grains." The truly best eggs to buy are the ones you get from your own chickens or from someone else who has chickens fed with grains and the chickens are outside running around. If you haven't eaten an egg from a chicken raised this way without all the hormones, antibiotics, and steroids, and fed with grains and which are outside, you are in for a treat. And if you eat the chicken raised this way, the taste is much better. You have to understand, it is all about money. They fatten the chickens up as quickly as possible, get them to the market pumped full of all kinds of things that are going to affect your health and wellbeing in a negative way and in many instances cause cancer. Again, big chicken manufacturers are not concerned with your health; they are all about selling chickens, diseased or not. There are not even enough inspectors to adequately oversee all the places that raise chickens.

If you were to visit a large chicken manufacturer and follow their assembly line as the chickens hang on hooks, you would see tumors in many of these chickens protruding out of their bodies. Next, you would see an employee take a knife and cut off—not out—the tumor where it is dropped in a bucket and mixed with antibiotics, growth hormones, and steroids among other things and mixed up and given to chickens as feed.

Stop smoking. This is probably the most difficult to do but the most rewarding in terms of money saved, better health, clearer thinking, less irritability, and a better attitude because you are not experiencing withdrawal symptoms. Foods will taste better because your taste buds are no longer anesthetized by nicotine. You will find you don't need all that salt you have been dumping on your foods just so you can taste them.

In about 2002 or 2003, I was conducting a "breathe-free" stop smoking seminar in Fort Morgan, Colorado. Not many people attended, but I was always excited when just one person would quit smoking. It was and is always a thrill to see how much happier they look and feel and excited they are when they have finally kicked the habit and addiction of nicotine.

One woman in particular who came was a registered nurse I worked with at the hospital. She was married and had a little boy. She was overweight, looked terrible, and I could tell she was unhappy, and she hated that she had a nicotine addiction. She finished the "breathe free" stop smoking seminar and I worked with her at the hospital and I remember she really struggled the first few weeks after the seminar, but she gained the victory and kicked the nicotine addiction. It wasn't long before I could see a big difference in the way she looked and in her attitude toward life. I don't remember how long after she quit smoking, maybe a few months, I just can't recall, but that she came up to me in surgery one day and said, "I'm so thankful I quit smoking." She told me she used to hide from her son when she smoked but now she doesn't have to hide anymore. She said, "That is just so good; I can be honest with my son for the first time."

Phillip Morris and other tobacco manufacturers don't care about people like this lady who was miserable and hated the day she smoked her first cigarette. They don't give a hoot that her nicotine addiction kept her away from her son when she wanted a cigarette for the first three years of his life. They love to see people, especially young people, who become addicted to nicotine. They don't care about anyone's health and well-being.

Cigarette smoke contains over 600 identified constituents. Here are just a few: acetaldehyde, alcohols, amides, ammonia, benzene, carbon monoxide, formaldehyde, hydrazine, hydrocyanic acid, hydrogen cyanide, insecticides, nicotine, nitric oxide, nitrosamines, polycyclic aromatic, hydrocarbons, toluene, and vinyl chloride. These ingredients make me think of a meth lab. Maybe you just need to add draino. These toxic substances increase your heart rate and blood pressure and drive up the demand for oxygen. Nicotine stimulates the adrenal gland directly (medulla) which secretes adrenaline and it affects our autonomic nervous system, which causes severe vasoconstriction, resulting in a reduction of blood flow to organs and tissues.

Just today, I was interviewing a patient who was scheduled for an elective ganglion cyst removal from her wrist. She told me she smokes one and a half pack of cigarettes a day. I asked her if she had any lung problems and she said, "No." But then I noticed on her list of medications that she was using an inhaler.

I then said, "I thought you said you don't have any lung problems."

She responded, "Well, sometimes it's difficult to breath and my chest will get tight and that's when I use my inhaler." I kindly informed her that her cigarettes were causing her chest tightness and difficulty in breathing. She said, "I know." I encouraged her to quit smoking. I also told her that nicotine was causing her heart rate to increase, causing her blood pressure to increase and the increase in heart rate was decreasing the rest cycle of the heart, and nicotine was causing a constriction of the coronary arteries in her heart, and that's what was contributing to her chest tightness.

When you breathe in fresh air or not so fresh air, depending on where you live, oxygen is carried to your organs and tissues and to every cell in your body by attaching itself to hemoglobin. Just think of hemoglobin as a train with many cars and each car is loaded with oxygen. The depot for this train is in your lungs where oxygen boards the train. That train then goes to the heart and is pumped throughout the entire body to every organ, muscle fiber, and every cell. This is where the oxygen gets off the train and nourishes every cell and brings healing to our mind, body, and soul. You can live without water for days, but in just a few minutes, you would die without oxygen. This is what is happening at the cellular lever in your body, especially in your lungs; cells are dying all the time when you are smoking.

I used to travel by train in the Amtrak back in the early 70's. We lived at that time in Michigan and I would board the train in Durand, Michigan, where there was a bustling train station at one time. My mother grew up in that area and she used the train to travel all over the country. Well, sometimes when I would be scheduled to board the train, many other people were also trying to get a ticket and so I didn't always get on board when I wanted to.

That's the way it is with oxygen trying to board the train of hemoglobin when you are smoking. Nicotine is competing with oxygen and carbon monoxide, which you are receiving from inhaling cigarette smoke and it has 200 times the affinity that oxygen has for hemoglobin that is responsible for carrying oxygen to the tissues and cells of your body. Consequently, the delivery of oxygen to the tissues throughout your body is greatly reduced. Oxygen's ability to be released is greatly impaired.

This is so important when it comes to healing. People who smoke have an up to 80 percent reduction in cellular healing. One of the worst-case scenarios for healing is to have an insulin dependent diabetic who smokes and has high blood pressure. I see it all the time in podiatry patients. The podiatrist schedules a patient for a wound debridement of a sore that will not heal on the foot. That patient sometimes will return again and again to have a little more of a toe or part of the foot removed until the whole foot and, yes, sometimes, the leg are amputated.

One final note on nicotine addiction. A relative new device known as the "hookah" (also known as a aheesha, nargile, or argileh), is a smoking device especially popular among teens and young adults. It is essentially a water pipe used to smoke flavored tobacco (virtually any flavor from chocolate to strawberry can be found) placed in the bowl at the top that is heated by charcoal, thus the user inhales charcoal residue as well. Sellers claim the smoke will be enjoyable and is smooth, producing heavy amounts of steam and smoke that can be exhaled as large, visible clouds. The "attributes" have great appeal to novice and youthful smokers. The health consequences of the hookah are misleadingly downplayed by both the manufacturers and merchants who supply them (Current Reviews for *Nurse Anesthetists*, Lesson 1, Volume 33, 5/23/2010.).

The hookah and more recently, the electronic cigarette, are now popular social activities especially among teens and young adults. There are hookah bars, restaurants, cafes, and dens.

The general belief, especially among young users, that hookahs are safer than cigarettes is incorrect. A recent article in JAMA, examining an FDA review of the electronic cigarette, notes that the device is just as toxic as a traditional cigarette.

The negative consequences of regular cigarette smoking can be applied to hookah and electronic cigarette users.

Again, the tobacco manufactures are focusing and targeting our children and youth to get them addicted to nicotine as early as possible. "The fox in charge of the hen house" takes on a whole new meaning.

This is the slice and dice of modern medicine. Very little in terms of lifestyle change is advanced to patients. Medicines are first prescribed and if that doesn't fix the problem—and most of the time it doesn't—then we have the knife. What is really sad to me is many of the patients I interview continue to smoke.

Just yesterday, I was talking with the young parents of a beautiful little eleven-month-old boy scheduled to have bilateral ear tubes placed. Knowing that a high percent of ear tubes are placed in very small children and infants because they are exposed to cigarette smoke, I said to the parents, "I would be remiss if I did not ask if either of you smoke?"

The father shook his head no and the mother quickly said, "I do, but I never smoke in the house or in the car with our baby there."

I told them that cigarette smoke is responsible for many of the ear tubes we place. I also told them that their baby is getting third hand smoke from the clothes she wears, from the upholstery in the car she rides in, and from the furniture in the house she lives in. Wherever her mother has been with her smoking, the baby will receive third hand smoke. I felt sorry for the mother who I knew was a little embarrassed over what I had told her even with all the empathy I could. Where is Phillip Morris and their high-paid executives when young people are suffering from the dastardly effects of their cigarette smoke?

Now do you think that Phillip Morris and many other tobacco companies don't know that these chemicals are in their tobacco? Of course, they do. Just a few years ago, Phillip Morris and other tobacco companies had to pay out some big fines. And who has been making commercials about quitting smoking? Surely not the tobacco companies who make the killer drug. Talk about putting the fox in charge of the hen house to kill even more hens; having tobacco companies in charge of making commercials and advertisements to help people stop smoking is surely a fitting description of that old adage. The last thing tobacco companies want you to do is stop smoking. There goes their profits down the toilet; but that is also where you will end up if you don't stop smoking.

I would be remiss if I didn't share with you how to kick the terrible addiction and habit of smoking cigarettes. Quitting is easy; but you may need some help and support to truly kick the habit. Someone said Mark Twain quit 2000 times.

The first thing I will always encourage everyone to do in making any lifestyle changes is begin a walking program. It is a non-impact exercise, doesn't cost you anything, and if you walk outside (which I strongly recommend), and breathe in deeply and slowly through your nose and out through your mouth, your attitude will actually change for the better.

Whenever you are making changes in your life, attitude is everything, especially when it comes to an addiction. It is all about mind over matter. Our Creator has placed within all of us a will and if we will exercise that will for good, it is the most powerful weapon we possess. Study the true nature of the will, which is your power to choose, because that's what your will is—the power of choice. It takes discipline. There is nothing more useless and weak than an undisciplined mind. In short, you discipline your mind by exercising your will; this is where your resolve to have victory in anything comes from. Does it take hard work? Yes, if you want to call sticking to something and persevering hard work.

First thing when you get up in the morning, say to yourself, "I love being free from smoking." That's a positive attitude and you have already started disciplining your mind for the battles that you will face throughout the day. You are already experiencing victory. Words are powerful, especially when you hear them repeated in the positive.

Victory for anything physical begins in the mind. If you say, "I can't lose weight, I can't stop smoking," you have already lost the battle. Feed into your mind positive thoughts, good thoughts, pure thoughts, noble thoughts and you will see and experience big changes in your life.

But words are only words if you don't take action and implement your words of positive affirmation. For many people, they love the taste of a cigarette when they first get up in the morning. You have to remember your blood levels of nicotine have dropped while you were sleeping and so your mind is telling your body to get some nicotine in here or I'm going to die; I'm starting to experience withdraw symptoms. Help!

Remember the diary you kept at the start of making lifestyle changes? Well, this would be a good time to keep a diary for a week while you are giving up nicotine. Make a list on a piece of paper and list in columns from left to right the number of cigarettes smoked, the time, the place, the activity before you smoked, was there an accomplice with whom you smoked, and the feelings you experienced after you smoked.

Make sure you note in your *stop smoking diary* the amount of money you saved by not smoking, because you will have more money immediately. Pretty soon, a pack of cigarettes and a gallon of gas are going to cost about the same. Now, the president of the United States may not care what a gallon of gas or a pack of cigarettes costs because he doesn't have to pay for either, but I guarantee the rest of America does care.

If you smoke, don't you want to get back control of your life? I did. At nineteen years old, I had smoked for about three years. In 1970, a pack of cigarettes didn't cost much; nor did a gallon of gas, but one day, I looked down at a cigarette I had placed between my fingers and I said, "I'm done smoking." I took the pack of non-filter Lucky Strikes and tore them up and I have never smoked again. Smoking is such a slavery and I want everyone who reads this book to be free again if they smoke. We have lost many more people from tobacco use than we ever did during the Civil War freeing Black people from slavery.

Here are some Short-Term Benefits of Smoking Cessation:

Within one week, taste and smell dramatically improve

- most physical withdrawal symptoms disappear
- fetus is free of nicotine
- teeth are whiter and mouth is fresher

Within one month, circulation improves

- blood platelets are activated
- respiratory problems decrease
- energy and stamina increase
- pulse rate and blood pressure lower
- hands and feet are warmer
- heart beat returns to normal
- stomach ulcer risk is minimized
- shortness of breath is reduced
- immune system is boosted
- skin color and tone are improved.

Some of the long-term benefits of smoking cessation are:

Chances of developing cancers of the pancreas, lungs, mouth, throat and esophagus, and cancers of the bladder, cervix, and larynx are all reduced.

In five to fifteen years after you quit smoking, "stroke risk" is reduced to that of a person who has never smoked.

Coronary heart disease and peripheral artery disease are cut in half within one year and after fifteen years of not smoking, you are as if you had never smoked.

Isn't that great news! We have been given amazing bodies and minds by our Creator to overcome almost every hereditary trait and tendency to self-destruction given to us through our genes from our parents or grandparents and from the polluted environment we may live in.

Drink plenty of pure water, at least six to eight glasses each day. Since you have quit smoking, you can treat yourself to some cool spring water. We take showers to clean the outside of our bodies and that feels so refreshing, especially if you alternate from hot to cold several times after you have finished showering; but we also need pure, clean, water on the inside. If we don't drink enough water, our blood becomes sluggish and that can leave us feeling run down and tired.

Thoreau once said, "Water is the only drink for a wise man." That statement has now been confirmed by the Adventist Health Study at Loma Linda University Medical Center. Jacqueline Chan, chief researcher on the project, said that sufficient water is as important to heart health as other factors such as diet, exercise, and abstinence from smoking. Healthy men who drank five or more glasses of water every day had a 54 percent decrease in the risk of fatal coronary heart disease compared with those who drank only two glasses of water. Women who drank five glasses of water lowered their fatal heart attack risk by 41 percent. Researchers believe that drinking a high volume of plain water works to thin the blood, thus lowering the risk of blood clots. People who replaced some of the water with other fluids, such as fruit juice, milk, or soda, did not receive the same protection."

"Five glasses of water will also decrease your risk of colon cancer by 45 percent, breast cancer by 79 percent, and bladder cancer by 50 percent."

Therese Allen, a quadriplegic, said she began drinking fourteen glasses of water each day after she suffered a serious kidney infection. Here's her story: "Talk about pain! I never wanted to go through that again. My doctor, however, told me that in my situation I could expect some kind of complication every two to four years. How could I prove this doctor wrong and avoid more infections? I decided to increase my water intake. Since that infection eighteen years ago, I've had the flu once, three colds, and only two infections. Water works!"

"But the sorry fact is that 75 percent of Americans are chronically dehydrated, and in 37 percent the thirst mechanism is so weak that it is often mistaken for hunger. Want to lose weight? Drink more water. Mild dehydration will slow down your metabolism as much as 3 percent. Lack of water is associated with daytime fatigue, back and joint pain, fuzzy short-term memory, trouble with basic math, and difficulty focusing on the computer screen or printed page." Kay Kuzma (*Morning Watch Book*)

Switching to a mostly liquid diet for the first twenty-four hours has many advantages. Change your routine associated with your smoking. Try pushing away from the dinner table right after you eat and take a little walk outside in the fresh air.

Eat plenty of fresh fruits and vegetables; this will aid in reducing the withdrawal symptoms you will experience. Fresh fruits and vegetables have been proven to be foods designed to prevent certain cancers, including lung cancers.

My anesthesia partner, Kevin Crawford, just today said something that is so true. He said, "Your food is your medication." He told me he eats one kiwi a day because it is about equal to taking a baby aspirin of 81mg a day as a blood thinner.

Kevin was pretty close to what the "Father of Medicine" Hippocrates wrote: "Let your food be your medicine and your medicine be your food."

I found an interesting quote on the internet written by Heather, a native Wisconsinite and Seattle transplant blogging about food. "America is one of the sickest nations on the planet. Despite our wealth, access to educational media, natural resources, and opportunity, most Americans accept atherosclerosis, cancer, hypertension, osteoporosis, heart disease, stroke, diabetes, and other degenerative chronic diseases as a part of the normal aging process."

Heather goes on to say: "Every single vitamin, mineral, and nutrient needed to grow and thrive is found in plants, fruits, vegetables, nuts, seeds, beans, and grains. And no you do not need cow's milk to get enough calcium."

"In fact, many green leafy vegetables have a calcium absorption rate of 50% while milk has only a 32% absorption rate."

"Everything I've ever studied about veganism supports it as a healthy way to eat and live. Have you ever heard of a medical report claiming that a vegan diet resulted in high blood pressure, diabetes, cancer or obesity? Of course not. Ever hear of a medical report claiming that a diet rich in meat and animal by-products would result in those ailments and more. Thought so."

Heather finishes with this paragraph: "You can be strong, muscular, athletic, and smart while eating vegan. There are some pretty famous and successful athletes that are vegan. Ever hear of Carl Lewis, winner of Olympic track medals? Or Tony Gonzales, the 247 pound member of the Kansas City Chiefs football team? UFC fighters...sure, Ricardo Moreira; body guilders? You bet...Robert Cheeke."

Right here I want to say something about the blood thinner, Plavix. It should be taken off the market. There is no test that the hospital lab can do to determine how soon your blood will clot after taking Plavix. It is a dangerous drug. If you're on Plavix, demand that your doctor find some other source to thin your blood. You need to be off Plavix a minimum of seven days before having surgery. The problem will come if you end up in the emergency room because of an accident and you are bleeding or you need to have emergency surgery, you could be at real risk of losing a lot of blood, if you have been on Plavix right up to the day of surgery.

Along with the six to eight glasses of pure fresh water you are drinking each day, add fresh frozen fruit juices (the sugar free kind). They are lower in calories, and will reduce withdrawal symptoms.

You may be saying at this juncture; what about alcohol instead all the fruit juices?

Alcohol weakens the resolve to remain smoke-free. Alcohol can remain in the brain especially in the frontal lobe of the brain where our reasoning center is located for up to two weeks. This is why guys like to get a girlfriend to drink a little alcohol; the girl is more apt to succumb to pressure from the guy to have premarital sex because her inhibitions have been weakened if not entirely removed.

Alcohol doubles risk of relapse and increases performance error, which leads to stress, which can lead to relapse; a vicious cycle is set up for failure when you are trying to stop smoking.

Alcohol suppresses the immune system, causing you to be even more susceptible to getting cancer.

Many times when you drink, you are socializing with friends and if they are smokers, the temptation may be too much for you not to take a cigarette when offered one.

Alcohol gives you a lot of empty calories and stimulates gastric juices, which increases appetite and now you have a desire to eat more. This is the very reason many young women have given me for not wanting to quit smoking; they are going to put on weight; but remember, ladies, you would have to almost become grossly obese to cause the same amount of damage to your body as cigarettes cause.

The alcohol and fermented wine industry do not care about your health in any way; they, along with the smoking industry, only care about making a profit. Every so often, I come across a study that touts the benefits of drinking some fermented wine each day. They say it protects the heart and that you will live longer and happier. I guess you might live happier if you're a happy drunk as was portrayed on the *Andy Griffith* show, but healthier, never. Where do you think these studies come from or at least who are the sponsors of these studies? You're right, it's the fermented wine and alcohol industry.

The benefits they are talking about in fermented wine that protects the heart come from the riboflavin and antioxidants that are found in fresh and wholesome grapes—without the fermentation found in fermented wine. What the studies don't reveal is the damage alcohol does to the other organs in your body and the financial disaster it can bring and the destruction of many families it causes.

One of the reasons I'm writing this book is to encourage people to get out of debt and get into health by making simple changes in their lifestyles. I just told my son last night about something that was occurring in his life that the right thing isn't always the easy thing to do, but the easy thing is usually the wrong thing to do.

Removing tobacco and alcohol from your life is a good place to start and you can accomplish both; you will be in better health and you will immediately have more money in your pocket. Just run the numbers. If you are a one-pack-a-day smoker and cigarettes are costing you five dollars a pack, then you will have thirty-five dollars more in a week, $140 more in a month, and $1,680 more in a year. If you smoke two packs a day, just double each of those figures and at the end of the year you will have $3,360.00 in your pocket. That is more than many people put away for retirement in a year. But the greatest savings isn't the money, it is your health; if you don't quit smoking, you need to worry about retirement. At the end of the day, do you think—as a smoker who never quit and now suffering from COPD, asthma, emphysema, or lung cancer and dragging around an oxygen tank—you will be saying, "I wish I would have smoked more; give me another unfiltered Lucky Strike or a Marlboro. I want to look like the cowboys that I see on the advertisements the tobacco giants use to lure unsuspecting people to get them addicted."

Trust me, my friends, these tobacco companies know very well once someone is addicted to nicotine, it will be *almost* impossible to quit smoking or dipping.

I don't know what alcohol costs because there are so many different ways you can buy it; but I know that it is expensive also, both financially and on your health. Because alcohol affects the frontal lobe of the brain, or the reasoning part of the brain, alcohol can bring financial ruin in just a very short time, especially if a person becomes an alcoholic. Accidents involving cars, buses, trains, and airplanes are becoming more frequent and can be directly linked and attributable to alcohol.

Chapter Six: Diabetes (Type 2 or Adult Onset)

Type 2 or adult onset diabetes is going to have to be renamed to include children. Type 2 diabetes is no longer just an adult disease. It is now affecting our children. There is probably two main reasons for this: One is inactivity, and the other is fats in the foods we consume. I'm amazed how many children I see eating at fast food places. Most children eat between meals and the greater percentage of the time what they eat between meals is junk food.

I can still remember watching *Leave It to Beaver* and when an episode showed Wally and Beaver coming into the house after school, their mom would be there to give them a glass of milk and some cookies; it was portrayed as something to tide them over until dinner and, of course, promoting milk.

For you to develop diabetes, two factors come in to play. The first is genetics, and the second is poor diet, a component of poor lifestyle.

This is one lifestyle disease that contributes to over 161,000 deaths each year, causes life expectancy to be shortened by six to nine years, and increases the risk for stroke and heart disease. So who wants to be a diabetic? Probably none of us, if we really think it through. Then why are over 600,000 new cases diagnosed each year? I believe the answer to that question is found in what is taught in terms of diabetes education.

Pharmaceutical companies are in business to make money and the way they make money is by selling drugs. In many of their advertisement deceptions, this is what is stated, "If diet and exercise isn't enough…," and then they go on to encourage the ingesting of one of their drugs for the rest of your life. As I have stated earlier, people want a quick fix to whatever is ailing them; most of us don't want to take the time or we don't think we have the time to exercise and eat differently. But if you don't take time to make changes in your lifestyle now, you may not be around to do it later.

Don't be one of the many that I see every day in the hospital who now have irreversible effects or damages from not taking the time to change their lifestyle early on in the areas of diet and exercise. What is really sad for me is when I see a family member—who didn't make lifestyle changes earlier—in ICU, clinging on for dear life.

There is no better investment you can make in your life than to get in health and stay in health by eating and drinking the right things and exercising and learning to cope with stress.

Frederick Banting, a Canadian scientist and co-discoverer of insulin said, "Insulin is not a cure for diabetes, it is a treatment. It enables the diabetic to burn sufficient carbohydrates, so that proteins and fats may be added to the diet in sufficient quantities to provide energy for the economic burdens of life."

When you have type 2 diabetes, high levels of sugar build up in your blood. This can lead to serious health complications. That's why controlling your blood sugar is key to managing diabetes. Keeping your blood sugar under control lowers your *risk for complications* later. High blood sugar can harm your organs and raise your risk of heart disease.

Having type 2 diabetes means that your body doesn't make enough insulin, or doesn't properly use the insulin your body makes. Insulin is a hormone made in your *pancreas*. It helps your body's cells use sugar (also called *glucose*), which comes from foods and drinks. Sugar is a source of energy for cells.

This book focuses on type 2 diabetes, the most common form of the disease. Typically, with type 2 diabetes, the body still makes insulin, but its cells can't use it. This is called *insulin resistance*.

Over time, high levels of sugar build up in the bloodstream. Being overweight and inactive increases the chances of developing type 2 diabetes.

Adult onset diabetes occurs through two factors: one is through genetics and the other is through diet. Most Americans are consuming the wrong diet every day. While the first, genetics, cannot be changed (that's what you were given in your suitcase when you came into this world), your diet can be changed. This is the beautiful thing. You and you only decide what you eat as an adult. You are the one in control of your lifestyle. You have to take back control of your lifestyle.

Last night, I just talked with a man who works on my car sometimes; he owns a successful repair shop. Recently, he had stents placed in his heart, not because he had a heart attack but because he had 98 percent and 97 percent blockage of his coronary arteries. He said after they placed the stents in his heart, he felt better, but last night, he said he is scheduled to return to Nashville to have more heart stents placed. His wife has high blood pressure and diabetes. I told him last night that I would love to help him make some changes in his lifestyle that could result in him and his wife feeling better. He doesn't need more stents; he desperately needs to make some lifestyle changes. Now, his heart disease and her diabetes may be too advanced to be completely reversed, but even so, some simple lifestyle changes may reduce their symptoms. They may even need to be on some of the medications prescribed to them for the rest of their lives but if they institute some simple lifestyle changes, they will be able to reduce the amount of medication they are consuming and reduce the symptoms they are experiencing. Oftentimes, the medications people are taking make them feel terrible.

Other main types of diabetes include:

Type 1 diabetes, which often affects children, although adults can develop it, too. In this form of diabetes, the body can't make insulin. The immune system mistakenly attacks the cells in the pancreas that make and release insulin. As these cells die, blood sugar levels rise. People with type 1 diabetes need insulin shots.

But even in this form of diabetes, instituting some simple lifestyle changes will help reduce the amount of insulin a person has to take. Just the other day I was doing a pre-anesthesia assessment on a patient scheduled for foot surgery; I had done her anesthesia for her last surgery, which lasted about six hours. I had to cancel her two weeks before that surgery because her blood sugar was out of control. She has an insulin pump and she usually can regulate her insulin very well. I asked her how long she has had diabetes, and she said since she was seven years old. She is now in her late thirties. I asked her if her parents have diabetes and she said no, and that no one, as far back as they could go in her family tree, had diabetes. But then she told me something very interesting. She said she has been doing research on the internet and she has discovered that a possible cause of her diabetes is when she received her MMR vaccination when she was six years old.

I read where autism is now possibly being linked to vaccinations because if you look at the time autism was discovered, vaccinations were being instituted. Coincidence? I don't think so. I have said and will continue to shout from the rooftop that drugs don't heal; they move around the symptoms that later pop up in some other place in the body. That's why if you continue on medications long enough, the doctor will place you on another medication to counteract the symptoms of the first medication; and so the viscous cycle repeats itself. I meet patients who are on as many as fifteen medications, sometimes more, and have been for years. They look miserable, feel miserable, and are miserable.

We need to get back to a plant-based diet. There is a book entitled *The China Study* and you can find it on the internet. I want to share a preface to that book here:

> One of the most comprehensive studies on nutrition ever done, *The China Study* provides us with some eye-opening information on how to lose weight and stay healthy and fit for life.
>
> *The China Study*, a massive nutrition research project that studied and analyzed the diets of more than 100 Chinese villages and how these diets correlate with heart disease, cancer diabetes, autoimmune disorders, macular degeneration, and

neurodegenerative diseases, is highly scientific, but very accessible and informative.

The findings of the book strongly favor a plant-based and whole-foods *diet*, which is counter to the Western diet which is typically high in fat, high in processed foods, and high in fat-laden meat. In fact, the authors of the book, father and son duo, Dr. Colin Campbell and Thomas Campbell, are vegans. But fear not, the *China Study* will not force you to never fry an egg again, but it will open your eyes to not just what we eat but the food industry that is responsible for making the food that ends up on our dinner table.

If you are at all interested in health, preventive disease, global health, food behaviors and how politics and the environment influence our food supply, *The China Study* is a must-read.

Arguments and Evidence

The China-Oxford-Cornell Study on Dietary, Lifestyle and Disease Mortality Characteristics in 65 Rural Chinese Counties, called in the book *The China Study*, was a comprehensive study of dietary and lifestyle factors associated with disease mortality in China, which compared the health consequences of diets rich in animal-based foods to diets rich in plant-based foods among people who are genetically similar.[3]

"Western" diseases correlated to concentration of blood cholesterol.

The China Study included a comparison of the prevalence of Western diseases (coronary heart disease, diabetes, leukemia, and cancers of the colon, lung, breast, brain, stomach, and liver) in each county. It was based on diet and lifestyle variables, and found that one of the strongest predictors of Western diseases was blood cholesterol with a statistical significance level equal to or exceeding 99.9 percent certainty. The study linked lower blood cholesterol levels to lower rates of heart disease and cancer. As blood cholesterol levels decreased from 170 mg/dl to 90 mg/dl, cancers of the liver, rectum, colon, lung, breast, leukemia, brain, stomach, and esophagus (throat) decreased. Rates for some cancers varied by a factor of 100 from those counties with the highest rates to the counties with the lowest rates.[5]

The authors write that "As blood cholesterol levels in rural China rose in certain counties, the incidence of 'Western' diseases also increased. What made this so surprising was that Chinese levels were far lower than we had expected. The average level of blood cholesterol was only 127 mg/dl, which is almost 100 points less than the American average (215 mg/dl).... Some counties had average levels as low as 94 mg/dl.... For two groups of about twenty-five women in the inner part of China, average blood cholesterol was at the amazingly low level of 80 mg/dl."[5]

Blood cholesterol levels correlated to diet, particularly animal protein.

The authors write that "Several studies have now shown, in both experimental animals and in humans, that consuming animal-based protein increases blood cholesterol levels. Saturated fat and dietary cholesterol also raise blood cholesterol, although these nutrients are not as effective at doing this as is animal protein. In contrast, plant-based foods contain no cholesterol and, in various other ways, help to decrease the amount of cholesterol made by the body." They write that "these disease associations with blood cholesterol were remarkable, because blood cholesterol and animal-based food consumption both were so low by American standards. In rural China, animal protein intake (for the same individual) averages only 7.1 grams per day whereas Americans average 70 grams per day."[6] They conclude that "The findings from the *China Study* indicate that the lower the percentage of animal-based foods that are consumed, the greater the health benefits—even when that percentage declines from 10 percent to 0 percent of calories. So it's not unreasonable to assume that the optimum percentage of animal-based products is zero, at least for anyone with a predisposition for a degenerative disease."[7]

Mechanisms of Action

Plants protect the body from disease, they argue, because many of them contain both a large concentration of and a large variety of antioxidants, which protect the body from damage caused by free radicals.[8] Western diseases are correlated with growth, which is associated with the increased risk of initiation, promotion and progression of disease, and that growth is correlated with a diet high in animal protein. They argue that the consumption of animal protein increases the acidity of blood and tissues and that to neutralize this acid, calcium (a very effective base) is pulled from the bones. They also state that higher concentrations of calcium in the blood inhibit the process by which the body activates Vitamin D in the kidneys to calcitriol, a form that helps regulate the immune system.

Misinformation about Nutrition

Campbell argues that "Most, but not all, of the confusion about nutrition is created in legal, fully disclosed ways and is disseminated by unsuspecting, well-intentioned people, whether they are researchers, politicians, or journalists," **and that there are powerful, wealthy industries that stand to lose a lot if Americans shift to a plant-based diet.**[9] Current studies on nutrition (specifically, the well-known *Nurses' Health Study*) are flawed, they argue, because they are overly focused on the effects of varying amounts of individual nutrients among individuals consuming a uniformly high-risk diet, including high levels of animal-based protein.[10]

Diseases Linked to Diet

Autoimmune Diseases

They argue that the risk of developing type 1 diabetes is strongly correlated with the consumption of cow's milk by infants.[11] Autoimmune diseases such as type 1 diabetes, multiple sclerosis, and rheumatoid arthritis have certain common features and may share the same cause or causes. They say that autoimmune diseases are more prevalent among people who live at higher geographic latitudes, and also among people who consume a diet high in animal protein, particularly cow's milk. They argue that Vitamin D is plausibly connected to both of these correlations. Vitamin D is important for the proper regulation of the immune system, and that for people who live at higher geographic latitudes, a lack of exposure to ultraviolet sunlight can result in a deficiency. The consumption of animal protein, especially casein, in cow's milk, results in higher concentrations of calcium in the blood, which inhibits the process by which the body activates Vitamin D in the kidneys to a form that helps repress the development of autoimmune diseases.[12]

Brain Diseases

They say that cognitive impairment and dementia, including Alzheimer's disease, are linked to hypertension, high blood cholesterol, and damage caused by free radicals, and that these risk factors can be controlled by diet.[13]

Cancer

The authors link breast cancer to long-term exposure to higher concentrations of female hormones, which in turn is associated with early menarche (age at first menstruation), late menopause, and a high concentration of blood cholesterol, and that all of these risk factors are linked to growth and a diet high in animal protein. The average Chinese woman is exposed to about 35-40 percent of the lifetime estrogen exposure of the average British or American woman, and that the rate of breast cancer among Chinese women is about one-fifth of the rate among Western women.[14]

They also argue that lower rates of colorectal cancer are associated with the consumption of plants high in fiber, such as beans, leafy vegetables, and whole grains.[8]

Diabetes

The authors describe a diet study conducted by James D. Anderson, M.D., of fifty patients—twenty-five with type 1 diabetes and twenty-five with type 2 diabetes—who were taking insulin to control their blood glucose concentrations. The authors reported that after these patients switched from the American-style diet recommended by the American Diabetes Association to a high-fiber, low-fat, plant-based diet, the patients with type 1 diabetes were able to reduce their insulin by an average of 40 percent within three weeks of changing their diet, and twenty-four of the twenty-five patients with type 2 diabetes were able to stop taking their insulin altogether within weeks.[15]

Eye Diseases

They argue that studies show a diet that includes carotenoids, which are found in colorful vegetables, provide protection from macular degeneration, an eye disease that can cause blindness, and that a diet that includes lutein, a particular antioxidant found in spinach, provides protection from cataracts.[16]

Heart Disease and Obesity

They say studies show that eating plant protein has a greater power to lower cholesterol levels than reducing fat or cholesterol intake.[13] At the time of their study, death rate from coronary heart disease was seventeen times higher among American men than rural Chinese men.[6] They write that "the average calorie intake per kilogram of body weight was 30 percent higher among the least active Chinese than among average Americans. Yet, body weight was 20 percent lower." The authors add that "consuming diets high in protein and fat transfers calories away from their conversion into body heat to their storage form as body fat (unless severe calorie restriction is causing weight loss.)" They argue that "diet can cause small shifts in calorie metabolism that lead to big shifts in body weight," adding that "the same low-animal protein, low-fat diet that helps prevent obesity also allows people to reach their full growth potential."[17]

Kidney Stones

The consumption of animal protein is linked to risk factors for the formation of kidney stones. They state that increased levels of calcium and oxalate in the blood may result in kidney stones, and that recent research shows that kidney stone formation may be initiated by free radicals.[18]

Osteoporosis

The authors state that osteoporosis is linked to the consumption of animal protein because animal protein, unlike plant protein, increases the acidity of blood and tissues. They add that to neutralize this acid, calcium (a very effective base) is pulled from the bones, which weakens them and puts them at greater risk for fracture. The authors add that "in our rural *China Study*, where the animal to plant ratio [for protein] was about 10 percent, the fracture rate is only one-fifth that of the U.S."

I place this information here about *The China Study* for you to understand that making simple lifestyle changes will not only add years to your life but also more productive and happy years. Many people are suffering with all kinds of diseases that they don't have to suffer from. I want to free as many people as I possibly can from the slavery of drug medications, television, inactivity, and unhealthful diets, as I can in the time I have left in my life.

If you are taking a lot of medications and were to enroll into one of the lifestyle centers I will list at the end of this book and go through their program, at the end of a month to six weeks, you would be off most of those medications; that's the NAKED TRUTH.

These lifestyle centers have been around for a long time and they all apply the eight laws of natural healing NEW-START (nutrition, exercise, water, sunshine, temperance, air, rest and trust in God).

Eight principles of food and health

The authors *of "The China Study"* describe their eight principles of food and health.[8]

1. **Nutrition represents the combined activities of countless food substances. The whole is greater than the sum of its parts.**
2. **Vitamin supplements are not a panacea for good health.**
3. **There are virtually no nutrients in animal-based foods that are not better provided by plants.**

4. **Genes do not determine disease on their own. Genes function only by being activated, or expressed, and nutrition plays a critical role in determining which genes, good and bad, are expressed.**
5. **Nutrition can substantially control the adverse effects of noxious chemicals.**
6. **The same nutrition that prevents disease in its early stages can also halt or reverse it in its later stages.**
7. **Nutrition that is truly beneficial for one chronic disease will support health across the board.**
8. **Good nutrition creates health in all areas of our existence. All parts are interconnected.**

"People who ate the most animal-based foods got the most chronic disease... People who ate the most plant-based foods were the healthiest and tended to avoid chronic disease. These results could not be ignored," said Dr. Campbell.

Gestational diabetes, which occurs in some pregnant women, can cause problems during pregnancy, labor, and delivery. Women who get gestational diabetes are more likely to develop type 2 diabetes.

In my practice of anesthesia, diabetes is one of the most crippling diseases I have to deal with. And what is amazing, type 2 diabetes can be completely eliminated through simple lifestyle changes, if caught early. That is the NAKED TRUTH. I meet people every day who tell me, "I'll always have type 2 diabetes because my father or my mother or my aunt had it."

But that just isn't true. Just because you came into this world through parents who had type 2 diabetes, or it was passed down to you from another relative doesn't mean that you have to suffer with type 2 diabetes for the rest of your life. Even if you inherited type 1 diabetes, you don't have to be on insulin for the rest of your life; if you institute some simple lifestyle changes you will be healthier for making those changes.

Drugs do not cure diabetes. If drugs cure diabetes, then why are so many people diabetics even after taking insulin or oral hypo-glycemics for years? Some people, when they are first diagnosed with diabetes because of their blood sugar levels, may need to be put on medications like oral hypo-glycemics or insulin for the short term, but certainly not for the rest of their lives, unless their disease has progressed too far.

My wife and I, our college-age daughter and her two college friends were vacationing in Sarasota, Florida, during our daughter's spring break. As I had to go to Wal-Mart for some items, I meandered over to the pharmacy section and for a moment looked up and saw two men standing at two pharmacy windows apparently waiting for a medication order to be filled. Both men appeared to be over sixty and maybe in their seventies. One man had about five or six medication bottles sitting on the counter. I stood there for over ten minutes watching those two men wondering if the medications they were waiting for were for themselves or for a family member. I thought to myself, *This is like cattle going to the slaughter house*. For some people, death would be welcomed over the effects of the drugs these people are taking, and mostly because they haven't changed their lifestyles. If patients were to really read the insert small print stating all the side effects, precautions, and warnings the pharmaceutical companies have to place on every drug container, because they know these drugs have the potential to hurt you and sometimes even kill you, patients would run away from taking most drugs.

"Although type 2 diabetes can be picked up by such blood tests for elevated sugar, many Americans do not seek out health professionals for such preventive services. They wait until they are sick. This is unfortunate. As a result, many type 2 diabetics only become aware of their disease when they experience potentially irreversible problems like eye or kidney disease, nerve problems, or they experience a heart attack."

Drugs on the whole may eliminate or at least alleviate the symptoms of a disease on the outside, but there may be hell to pay on the inside. Remember, all these drugs work at the cellular level in our bodies. The body on the inside and on the outside is made up of trillions of cells either tightly or loosely packed together. Any medication you take, whether you take it through your vein or intramuscularly, through an inhaler, or by applying a cream or ointment topically, or subcutaneously, they all work at the cellular level.

Treating the symptoms of the disease instead of treating the disease itself by changing your lifestyle is like a doctor and nurse called to a treatment room where they find water covering the entire floor. They can see a water pipe has burst under the sink, but instead of repairing the broken water pipe or calling for a plumber, they are mopping the floor up with mops in their hands and wringing the water out into a bucket. We have to get at the root cause of the disease which most of the time is associated with our lifestyle. If you keep just treating the symptoms and not the root of the problem, you are going to feel and look like that wrung out mop.

You may feel better almost immediately after taking some form of medication or drug, but what is the lasting affect? Most of the time, it is because our blood level of that drug has fallen low enough to trigger withdrawal symptoms, so after taking the drug, our blood level of that drug is elevated and presto, we feel better or so we think. It is just like drinking a cup of coffee or soft drink that has caffeine. You might at first feel more alert or awake or energized, but the ultimate result will be a downer. At the end of the day after consuming coffee and soft drinks, you just feel washed out. *What is that drug doing on the inside of my body at the cellular level?* is the most important thing to consider. The reason I use the words "medication and drug" is I believe there is a difference between the two—a big difference.

A medication is something you take that can actually aide in the healing process at the cellular level. For instance, when someone has a ruptured appendix, we administer an antibiotic and usually more than one. Why? If the bacteria attacking us on the inside are not eliminated, the body's ability to begin the healing process may be overwhelmed. That doesn't mean without antibiotics, the body cannot heal itself. But many times, because of the lifestyle of the individual, i.e. obesity, diabetes, hypertension, alcohol, and nicotine use, the body's ability to heal is greatly diminished. So a medication given in conjunction with some changes in a person's lifestyle can prove to be beneficial. But we must remember where true healing comes from. It doesn't come from the antibiotics. It comes from the Great Physician—our Creator, God.

On the other hand, a drug may start out to be a medication if used to control symptoms in the short term while a person begins making simple lifestyle changes. But it becomes a drug when used chronically to treat a disease without that individual making some changes in lifestyle. Will some people have to be on medication for the rest of their lives? Maybe, but the amount of medication needed will be greatly reduced when taken in conjunction with lifestyle changes.

One of the most overrated surgeries of my lifetime is open-heart surgery to remove blockage of plaque buildup in the coronary arteries—those arteries that bring life-giving oxygen to the heart muscle—for without your coronary arteries, you would die. In lay terms, this surgery is referred to as a "CABG", pronounced cabbage. In medical language, it is "Coronary Artery Bypass Graft." What's interesting about this whole scenario is if the patient were to institute some immediate lifestyle changes by eating simple foods, become vegetarians, at least for the short term, get between seven and nine hours of sleep a night, and start exercising first by walking, they would not even need to have open heart surgery. Now, some people have done this before their scheduled surgery, and they are already feeling better, but the doctor has convinced them that because they have had an MI or they have 90-100 percent blockage in their coronary arteries, they must have heart surgery now. Nothing could be further from the truth. The NAKED TRUTH is that if after discovering you have major coronary blockage or have experienced an MI, and you make lifestyle changes in your eating, sleeping and exercise, you will not need heart surgery. For the most part a CABG is a SHAM surgery and just add the letter "e" to the word sham and you have "SHAME." Yes, it's a shame for people to have to go through a surgery of this magnitude, when changing their lifestyle is the only treatment they need; and, lifestyle changes would have prevented the blockage and an MI.

At the end of my book, you will find a list of lifestyle treatment centers that I highly recommend.

Pharmaceutical companies cannot make any money if you implement simple lifestyle changes. They would like to bring under their control all herbal treatments, many of these herbs you can grow in your own back yard.

It can take years to build up the kind of plaque in your coronary arteries that will cause an MI or result in 90-100 percent blockage; and, remember, exercise doesn't remove plaque from your arteries. Plaque is removed by changing the foods we eat.

I remember traveling out west years ago when one of the main thoroughfares was completely blocked because of a mudslide. The highway was completely closed. No traffic could get by or through all the debris that cluttered the road. The highway department had already in place other roads that allowed the traffic to get around the blocked road so travelers could reach their destinations, maybe not on time, but finally arrive safely. That is the way our body works. Over the years, the body develops what we call in medicine collateral circulation. That is, when you have a vein stripping done, say, on your lower legs, and they remove your saphenous vein, your body already has other veins to get blood through or around the missing or obstructed vein. Well, the same is true with the coronary arteries. As our coronary arteries become partially or completely obstructed with plaque, over the years, other arteries have developed that supply blood to our heart muscle—but not as effective as the coronary arteries we were born with. When a patient presents to the ER complaining of chest pain and has had an MI or has a partial or complete blockage of their coronary arteries, the reason that person isn't dead already is because of collateral circulation; he or she can be thankful for his or her gene pool. Over the years, he or she has developed a collateral circulation. After receiving some acute care at the ER for chest pain, if that patient immediately puts in place some simple lifestyle changes, they will not have to have a CABG. In an acute crises, we would administer Morphine, nitroglycerine, aspirin, and give supplemental oxygen. These are all good medicines to administer and hopefully they will not be for long-term treatment.

Nitroglycerine (NTG) dilates the coronary arteries and relieves the coronary spasms the person may be experiencing, and consequently your heart muscle receives more oxygen. The lack of oxygen to the heart muscle is what's causing the severe chest pain.

There are people walking around who have been prescribed NTG to take if they experience chest pain. If after taking NTG three times and they are still experiencing chest pain, they have been instructed to go to the emergency room ASAP. Well, guess what, there are people who are taking NTG tablets like some people chomp down Tums with no plan for changing their lifestyles.

When I interview patients who are going for surgery, I always ask them if they are on any kind of blood thinners, i.e. Plavix, Coumadin, or aspirin. Many times, they will say, "I'm taking aspirin." I ask them, "Why are you on aspirin?" and many times they'll say, "My doctor told me I needed to." Years ago, I administered anesthesia for a general surgeon who at the time was forty-seven years old. He told me he was taking aspirin every day—a baby Aspirin, 81 mg. He said his doctor said it would help prevent a stroke; so, like an ox to the slaughter, goes this poor doctor.

Readers, aspirin is not an innocuous drug. It will eat the tender lining of your stomach mucosal. Many of my patients are taking aspirin as an anticoagulant. I know many doctors that are taking aspirin. I asked a doctor recently why he was taking aspirin-81mg every day; he said, "My doctor told me I should be on it as a safeguard against stroke. This doctor had no medical issues, was forty-six years of age and was not taking any other medications. That is absolutely asinine.

One kiwi a day will give you the anticoagulant ability that a baby aspirin of 81mg will give you. Oh, yes, I almost forgot, the drug cartels cannot produce kiwi in a pill form—yet. Many times, doctors are puppets of the pharmaceutical companies and they just dispense pills like candy just because the drug cartels have some biased study financed that says aspirin will help prevent strokes. But if you take the time to read the fine print on the precautions about aspirin, hopefully you will never take it.

Some people do not develop this collateral circulation and if their coronary arteries become completely or even partially blocked, they can die. It's what we call sudden death. There is no resuscitation with these people. It's over, lights out, curtain time, the play is over. My older brother was one of those sudden death statistics at the age of forty-two. Last year, his oldest son died at the age of forty on Christmas eve; and his next son has experienced two MI's already; he is only thirty-eight. With my brother and his two sons, both lifestyle and genetics played a role in their early demise; but I believe lifestyle was the biggest factor.

The following is a quote from my all-time favorite author on health and happiness who wrote this over one hundred years ago. The road to health really hasn't changed. The basic principles and tenets of good living remain the same. There are a lot more turn offs on the road to health. But the road to health itself is paved with common sense through simple lifestyle changes.

"Many transgress the laws of health through ignorance, and they need instruction. But the greater number know better than they do. They need to be impressed with the importance of making their knowledge a guide of life. The physician has many opportunities both of imparting a knowledge of health principles and of showing the importance of putting them into practice. By right instruction, he can do much to correct evils that are working untold harm {MH 126.1}.

A practice that is laying the foundation of a vast amount of disease and of even more serious evils is the free use of poisonous drugs. When attacked by disease, many will not take the trouble to search out the cause of their illness. Their chief anxiety is to rid themselves of pain and inconvenience. So they resort to patent nostrums (quack medicine) of whose real properties they know little, or they apply to a physician for some remedy to counteract the result of their misdoing, but with no thought of making a change in their unhealthful habits. If immediate benefit is not realized, another medicine is tried, and then another. Thus the evil continues {MH 126.2}.

People need to be taught that drugs do not cure disease. It is true that they sometimes afford present relief, and the patient appears to recover as the result of their use; this is because nature has sufficient vital force to expel the poison and to correct the conditions that caused the disease. Health is recovered in spite of the drug. But in most cases, the drug only changes the form and location of the disease. Often, the effect of the poison seems to be overcome for a time, but the results remain in the system and work great harm at some later period {MH 126.3}.

By the use of poisonous drugs, many bring upon themselves lifelong illness, and many lives are lost that might be saved by the use of natural methods of healing. The poisons contained in many so-called remedies create habits and appetites that mean ruin to both soul and body. Many of the popular nostrums called patent medicines, and even some of the drugs dispensed by physicians, act a part in laying the foundation of the liquor habit, the opium habit, the morphine habit, that are so terrible a curse to society {MH 126.4}.

The only hope of better things is in the education of the people in right principles. Let physicians teach the people that restorative power is not in drugs, but in nature. Disease is an effort of nature to free the system from conditions that result from a violation of the laws of health. In case of sickness, the cause should be ascertained. Unhealthful conditions should be changed, wrong habits corrected. Then nature is to be assisted in her effort to expel impurities and to re-establish right conditions in the system {MH 127.1}.

Natural Remedies

Pure air, sunlight, abstemiousness, rest, exercise, proper diet, the use of water, trust in divine power—these are the true remedies. Every person should have a knowledge of nature's remedial agencies and how to apply them. It is essential both to understand the principals involved in the treatment of the sick and to have a practical training that will enable one rightly to use this knowledge {MH 127.2}.

The use of natural remedies requires an amount of care and effort that many are not willing to give. Nature's process of healing and up building is gradual, and to the impatient, it seems slow. The surrender of hurtful indulgences requires sacrifice. But in the end it will be found that nature, untrammeled, does her work wisely and well. Those who persevere in obedience to her laws will reap the reward in health of body and health of mind {MH 127.3}.

Too little attention is generally given to the preservation of health. It is far better to prevent disease than to know how to treat it when contracted. It is the duty of every person, for his own sake, and for the sake of humanity, to inform himself in regard to the laws of life and conscientiously to obey them. All need to become acquainted with that most wonderful of all organisms, the human body. They should understand the functions of the various organs and the dependence of one upon another for the healthy action of all. They should study the influence of the mind upon the body, and of the body upon the mind, and the laws by which they are governed {MH 128.1}.

We cannot be too often reminded that health does not depend on chance. It is a result of obedience to law. This is recognized by the contestants in athletic games and trials of strength. These men make the most careful preparation. They submit to thorough training and strict discipline. Every physical habit is carefully regulated. They know that neglect, excess, or carelessness, which weakens or cripples any organ or function of the body, would ensure defeat {MH 128.2}.

The power of the mind is incredible. I found a few more paragraphs written over a hundred years ago and applicable today:

Those who will gratify their appetite, and then suffer because of their intemperance, and take drugs to relieve them, may be assured that God will not interpose to save health and life which is so recklessly periled. The cause has produced the effect. Many, as their last resort, follow the directions in the Word of God, and request the prayers of the elders of the church for their restoration to health. God does not see fit to answer prayers offered in behalf of such, for He knows that if they should be restored to health, they would again sacrifice it upon the altar of unhealthy appetite.

There is a call of invalids who have no real located disease. But as they believe they are dangerously diseased, they are in reality invalids. The mind is diseased, and many die who might recover of disease, which exists alone in the imagination. If such could have their minds diverted from themselves, from noticing every poor feeling, they would soon improve. Inactivity will cause disease. And to this the indulgence of unhealthy appetite, and drug-taking, and those who had no real located disease will become invalids in very deed. They make themselves so. If such would engage in cheerful, healthy labor, they would rise above poor feelings. Even if they should become very weary at times, it would not hurt them. As they would accustom themselves to healthy, active labor, the mind would be occupied, and not find time to dwell upon every ache and pain.

If invalids would dispense with medicines of every description, improve their habits of eating, and exercise as much as possible in the open air, their names would soon be dropped from the invalid list. The power of the will is a mighty soother of the nerves, and can resist much disease simply by not yielding to ailments and settling down into a state of inactivity. Those who have but little force and natural energy need to constantly guard themselves, lest their minds become diseased and they give up to supposed disease, when none really exists. It is slow murder for persons to confine themselves, days, weeks, and months in doors, with but little outdoor exercise.

The above statement reminds me of Howard Hughes and the recluse he became and how it affected his health. The mind is powerful and if you reset your mindset, you can accomplish just about anything you desire.

Sometimes, as an anesthesia provider, I am called to administer I.V. sedation to a patient whose heart rate is extremely fast; this, after the doctor has tried medication and now would like to perform cardioversion (restoring the rhythm of the heart to normal by applying direct-current electrical shock). This is what happens when we reset our mindset—we return to the original lifestyle our Creator gave us.

Here is the beauty of changing how we think. You really can't have great physical health without first having good mental health. If you improve your thinking—and you can—by habit and by accustoming yourself to cheerful reflection, your physical health will improve. A force will be imparted to the lifesprings, the blood will not move sluggishly, as would be the case if you were to yield to despondency and gloom. Your mental and moral health are invigorated by the buoyancy of your spirits. The power of the will can resist impressions of the mind and will prove a grand soother of the nerves.

We have an incredible defense system built into our minds but we have to choose to use it. I heard a neurosurgeon say that the brightest minds only use 10-15 percent of their brains.

Others are too active in body and mind. The mind of such must rest as well as the body, and without it, will be overworked, and the constitution must break down. Satan exults to see the human family plunging themselves deeper and deeper into suffering and misery. He knows that persons who have wrong habits and unsound bodies cannot serve God so earnestly, perseveringly, and purely as though sound. A diseased body affects the brain. With the mind, we serve the Lord. The head is the capitol of the body. If the finger is pricked, the nerves, like telegraphic wires, bear the intelligence immediately to the brain. Satan triumphs in the ruinous work he causes by leading human families to indulge in habits that destroy themselves and one another; for by this means he is robbing God of the service due Him.

In order to preserve health, temperance in all things is necessary: temperance in labor, temperance in eating and drinking. Because of intemperance, a great amount of misery has been brought upon the human family. The eating of pork has produced scrofula (primary tuberculosis of the lymphatic glands, especially those of the neck.

Pork eating is still causing the most intense suffering to the human race. Depraved appetites crave those things that are most injurious to health. The curse, which has rested heavily upon the earth and felt by the whole race of mankind, has also been felt by the animals. The beasts have degenerated in size and length of years. They have been made to suffer more than they otherwise would by the wrong habits of man.

There are but a few animals that are free from disease. They have been made to suffer greatly for want of light, pure air, and wholesome food. When they are fattened, they are often confined in close stables and are not permitted to exercise and have free circulation of air. Many poor animals are left to breathe the poison of filth left in barns and stables. Their lungs will not long remain healthy while inhaling such impurities. Disease is conveyed to the liver, and the entire system of the animal is diseased. They are killed and prepared for the market, and people eat freely of this poisonous animal food. ***Much disease is caused in this manner***. But people cannot be made to believe that it is the meat they have eaten that has poisoned their blood and caused their sufferings. Many die of diseases caused wholly by meat-eating, yet the world does not seem to be the wiser.

These health principles stated above were written over a hundred years ago. General health principles do not change. It is what our grandparents and great grandparents were doing; they were living out the basic health principles. Pharmaceutical companies (legal drug cartels) would have you believe you can't have good health without first being on one of their drugs. Also, I want to say a word here about vitamin and herbal conglomerates. These are also billion-dollar businesses that don't always have your best interest at heart because, for the most part, vitamin and herbal manufacturers are not regulated by the FDA as are pharmaceutical companies. Many people have no idea what the herbs and vitamins are doing to their bodies and minds.

Years ago, I read an article in the *Readers' Digest* entitled, "Americans Have the Richest Urine in the World": Because Americans were consuming mega doses of vitamins and paying a premium price for them and most of those vitamins were excreted in the urine, Americans had the richest urine in the world.

Vitamins do have their place, especially in Third World countries where there are not enough fruits and vegetables available. Even here in America, people, especially children, who are eating out a lot at fast food restaurants, may need vitamin supplements. But if you are eating a variety of fresh fruits and vegetables, you will receive all the vitamins you'll ever need.

Every day I see new ads on how to live healthier lives and how to lose weight, and they all have something to sell. Most of these ads will give you the first thirty-day supply free. They purport that if you take their little capsule, pill or even eat this or that one thing, you will start losing weight immediately or whatever else they claim it will do.

Don't fall for those ads. They are nothing more than health scams. The single most important key to good health is balance and moderation and temperance in everything we do and eat. Getting back to a plant-based diet and away from a meat-based diet is the key.

What's interesting is that if we took all the grains being grown to feed and fatten animals to eat, and instead gave them to people to eat, hunger in this world as we know it would be wiped out. This week even as I am writing this book, thousands of people have been killed and many more are presumed dead by the deadliest earthquake to hit Japan in decades. It measured 8.9. Thousands of people are without food and water and the very basics of ever day life that we take for granted in America. Instead of trying to get meat over to them to eat, we could send grains and rice and fruits and vegetables at much less cost and they would do much better.

Diseases of the "affluent," like heart disease, stroke, and cancer come largely from the consumption of diseased meat. When you go to the grocery store and step up to the meat section and see a sign that says freshly packaged meat, some of that meat has been freshly packaged but only after cutting out the spoiled parts. Many times, that's the same meat that was there decaying yesterday. Nothing is going to be wasted when it comes to selling dead carcasses. It cost too much to get it there.

If you are a vegetarian or you want to become a vegetarian, I have included this next article from the internet for you. Not many people understand how many foods contain gelatin; but if you are a purist, you need this information.

If you want to use gelatin to thicken things up, you can buy vegan gelatin at a health food store. My wife gets vegan gelatin from the village market in Collegedale, Tennessee.

I found an article on the internet from Buzzle.com-Home Topics Latest Articles about gelatin ingredients.

Gelatin Ingredients

Gelatin ingredients can never be vegetarian! What exactly are the constituents of gelatin? Presented below is more information on gelatin, its ingredients and uses.

Gelatin, also known as gelatin, is a colorless water-soluble protein. The jelly used in most desserts and sweets is made of gelatin. Gelatin in its natural form is colorless, odorless, and tasteless. There have been many conceptions, misconceptions, and beliefs about ingredients in gelatin. Let us have a look at it in detail.

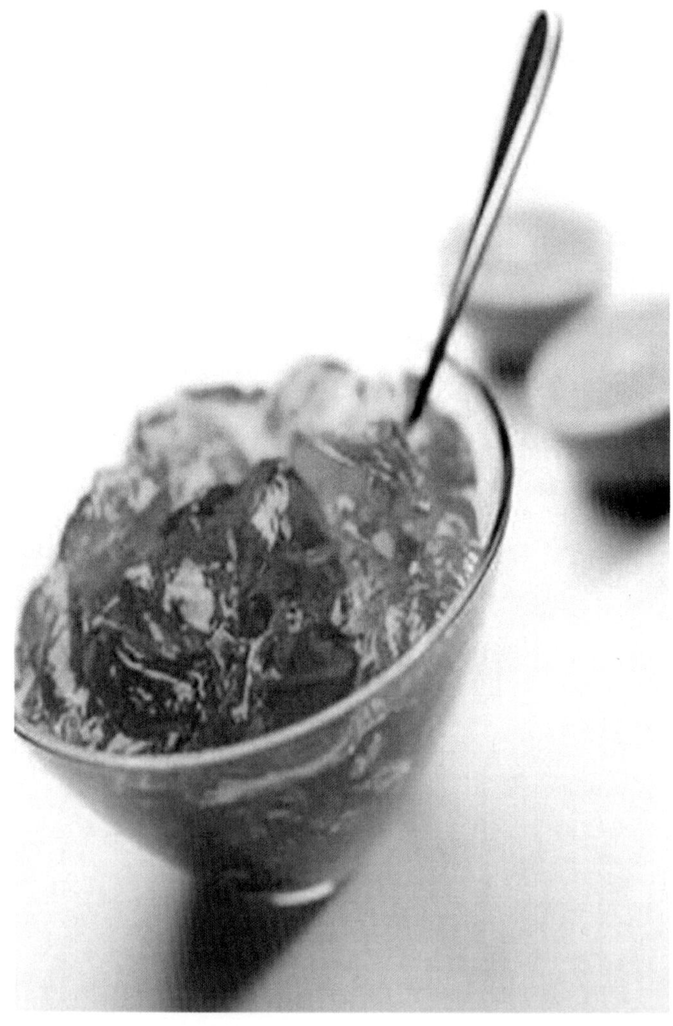

Gelatin Ingredients

Collagen is one of the chief ingredients of gelatin. Collagen is a scleroprotein found in the bone, cartilage and tendons of animals. When the bones or tissues of animals are boiled, collagen yields gelatin. Hence, getting straight to the point, you should know that gelatin can be obtained only from animal tissues. There is a widespread misconception that gelatin is obtained from horse hooves, which is incorrect. Horse hooves or bones are never used in the production process of gelatin. Tissues of pigs, cattle, and fish are prominently used in order to obtain gelatin.

Therefore, it is no doubt clear that as gelatin is gotten from animal sources, it cannot be considered as a *vegetarian meal* or product. Similarly, any product containing gelatin, like marshmallows, gummy bears, Peeps, Jell-O, etc. can never be included in vegan food products. Many capsule covers are also made with gelatin and hence, vegetarians should specifically have a check at the label of any medicine to make sure whether they are vegetarian or not. Gelatin is also one of the chief ingredients of toothpaste, certain cosmetics, and soups and canned hams. Gelatin is commonly available in the form of granules, flakes, as well as cubes.

Kosher Gelatin

The answer to the query, 'Is Kosher gelatin vegan or not?' is very ambiguous. Kosher or Kashrut, are a set of rules followed by the Jewish community about the production and edibility of food products. According to Kosher laws, any food items that contain flesh are considered as non-kosher while those gotten from plants are considered as kosher. However, as gelatin is obtained from bones and not from actual flesh, it is considered as kosher and can be eaten by Jewish adherents. Secondly, only gelatin that comes from fish and all types of vegetarian gelatin are considered kosher. However, it is always advisable to check Kosher laws and gelatin ingredients thoroughly before consuming any of such products.

Vegan Gelatin

Vegans may be disappointed to find that gelatin used in their favorite desserts is obtained from an animal source and hence, cannot be consumed. One should also know that no such product as the vegan gelatin exists. However, one may not be aware, but there are substances that have similar properties to that of gelatin and can be used as a substitute to it. Agar agar, or only agar, is a widely used vegan substitute for gelatin. Agar is obtained from seaweed or red algae and is used as an ingredient in many vegan desserts all over the world. Agar is obtained by boiling, purifying, and drying red algae or red seaweed. The properties of agar are not exactly similar to that of gelatin, as it is more slimy and softer than gelatin. But nonetheless, it makes an excellent gelling agent in vegan marshmallows and jellies. Some of the other vegan substitutes for gelatin include Xanthan, Biobin, Guar, and Carob fruit.

If you're confused about the same, refer to the food guide.

Now that you are aware of gelatin ingredients, it is always advisable to check the label of every product, especially desserts or canned foodstuffs. Presence of gelatin in it means it has been prepared from an animal source, which definitely is not a vegan option!

By Madhura Pandit

Published: 3/6/2010

Why is it that not much is being said about these things? Because America has gone amuck with political correctness. We are almost in a mad frenzy in the opposite direction making sure that someone doesn't say something that might offend someone else. But the NAKED TRUTH is thousands of people are dying every single day directly and indirectly from all the DRUGS they are consuming. First lady Michelle Obama has been attacked for trying to make sure people are eating better and exercising more. I don't know her personally, but I believe her intentions are honorable. She definitely could have taken on some other issue that would not have stirred up such a hornet's nest; but she didn't and that's why I support her. No, I don't believe the government should or even can legislate and definitely cannot enforce what foods people consume or the way they live their lives. But when it comes to being insured and receiving medical treatment, I really believe those who are living healthier lifestyles should have HUGE insurance discounts as opposed to those who are not.

What about those patients admitted to the hospital for surgery with severe COPD from smoking all their lives, or the patients who are grossly obese from out of control eating and lack of exercise? Should other people who make decisions to eat better and exercise more and not smoke or drink not be given preferential treatment and receive large discounts from insurance companies?

Just last Friday, I interviewed a woman in her forties who was having a laparoscopic cholecystectomy surgery; the surgeon was going to remove her gallbladder. She weighed 340 pounds, was 5 feet 2 inches tall and had no neck; her head sat right on her shoulders like the snowballs of a snowman fit together. After taking a history, I informed her that she was at increased risk of going under a general anesthetic because of all her extra adipose tissue. She asked, "What's that?"

I frankly said, "That is fat." As I always try to do with my patients, I share with those who really need to make lifestyle changes how to go about doing that. Of course, I told her she needed to lose weight and some simple things she could do that wouldn't cost her a penny; in fact, it would save her money. This patient really didn't need her gallbladder removed. She didn't have gallstones. She only had some cholecystitis or inflammation of the gallbladder. There was nothing life-threatening about her gallbladder being inflamed and with the right lifestyle changes implemented, she could probably keep her gallbladder. About 80 percent of all gallstones are made up of cholesterol. The sad part for many patients I interview for other surgeries who have had their gallbladder removed is when they say, "Since I have had my gallbladder taken out, I can eat all kinds of foods that used to give me excruciating pain." So the good surgeon has removed one of the alarm systems set up in the body as a warning for us when we may be eating the wrong foods.

Almost everyone who has type 2 or adult onset diabetes has eaten their way to that diagnosis along with a lack of exercise.

The Naked Truth is you can literally eat your way back to health; I mean, if you like to eat that sounds like fun.

The reason we are not diagnosed with diabetes, hypertension, and many other diseases until later in life is we have ignored or haven't understood good health practices. It usually takes years of neglect to run down the complex creation of the human body and mind. The old saying of "mind over matter" has real meaning when it comes to making changes in our lifestyles.

Diseases that are primarily the result of wrong lifestyle choices usually take a while for symptoms to develop "operating or proceeding in an inconspicuous or seemingly harmless way but actually with grave effect: an insidious disease."

Years ago when I was still doing stop smoking seminars or smoking cessation programs—they were later named breathe free seminars—I would now and then have somebody come up to me on opening night of the seminar and say, "So you're the one who is going to get me to stop smoking." I would always reply to this comment, "No, you are going to stop and I am going to show you how to keep from starting up again." I always tell people quitting smoking is easy, Mark Twain quit 2000 times, but staying off tobacco is something quite different,.

Good ole Abe said it well: "You can't help men permanently until they help themselves." This is why changing your lifestyle is so important. You take back control of your life. If you obey the laws of health, you will be happier, healthier, wiser, and more prosperous.

And these principles or basics to good health haven't changed since the Good Lord created us some six thousand years ago. The human machinery is still as complex as it was the moment God breathed into our nostrils the breath of life and we became a living soul.

The biggest problem with diabetes is poor circulation, which increases infection and slows healing. I can't tell you how many patients I administer anesthesia to for foot surgeries that have diabetes. No one wants to have a foot amputated. But many times, we start out with amputating a toe, then another toe and another and then a portion of the foot, and sometimes the whole foot, and yes, rarely the lower leg but it does happen. We call this "peace mill" surgery, one peace at a time. And rarely do I see much emphasis placed on making simple lifestyle changes. This is the finest in allopathic medicine, drugs and surgery, drugs and surgery, until the patient welcomes death as opposed to a miserable existence of the knife and drugs. Why do you think that drug addicts feel so miserable? This is a billion-dollar industry. Doctors, for the most part, know patients want a quick fix; they know if they don't give them something that will help right away, the patients are going to go down the street to another physician who will oblige them with the latest drug or surgical intervention; and if that doctor is an hospital paid employee, he better see all the patients he can or he will be out of work at the hospital.

I recently was told the story of an American man who, while working in China, got sick and had symptoms of tonsillitis. He made an appointment to see a doctor. The doctor confirmed his diagnosis of tonsillitis. The man said, "Well, I'm going back to America and have my tonsils removed." The doctor informed him he didn't need to have his tonsils removed: He would give him some herbs and he would get well. The man followed the doctor's advice and got well. The doctor also told the American, "We get paid to not admit people to a hospital. In America, it is just the opposite; doctors get paid to admit people to a hospital. It's all about money; the NAKED TRUTH is hospitals don't really care about you as much as they do your money.

A lot of people who have diabetes in the extreme, who have lost a toe, a foot, a leg, or who are on weekly dialysis, are also on some form of an antidepressant.

You have to understand, for hospitals and outpatient surgery centers, it is all about numbers. Many doctors now are employed by hospitals; but that is actually a conflict of interest. The hospital tells the doctor, "You must meet a quota of patients each month; otherwise, the hospital is losing money paying your salary." Just recently, I was eating lunch with our orthopedic surgeon who is employed by the hospital and is seventy-three years of age; and so although he needs to work, he doesn't want to overwork. He became a hospital employee so he wouldn't have to work so hard. He told me that the CEO of our hospital had met with him for lunch one day last week and had said, "We are losing $10,000.00

a month paying your salary; we need more cases from you in surgery." The CEO also told this orthopedic surgeon, "What I care about are numbers, because numbers represents money and without money you don't get paid and I can't keep the operating staff we need."

With the healthcare industry in shambles, we are going to see more and more doctors becoming hospital employees. Why? Money and control. CEO's of hospitals and surgery centers don't care about your health. If you have good insurance or the independent wealth to pay for medical and hospital care, they would like to have you as a frequent flyer. And in conjunction with the drug cartels (pharmaceutical companies), they would love to see you being treated for hypertension, diabetes, GERD, obesity, depression, and taking medications for all these diseases and having surgeries, but they really don't want you cured. This is especially true with the drug cartels. If you are cured, you no longer need any of their life-destroying drugs. It is a vicious cycle in the medical community today, treating patients with drugs followed by surgery.

There is a time for using medications. I didn't call them drugs, because when used properly and for the most part temporarily, they can aid in healing. But I interview patients going to surgery everyday who are on a long list of drugs, not medications, and healing is not taking place. If healing isn't taking place, they are using drugs—but if we are not getting any place with slam dunking you with drugs, we have the knife and we'll take you to surgery and destroy you piece by piece, limb by limb, organ by organ until you're left a miserable wreck of humanity. If I were diagnosed with a terminal illness, I would rather go to the mountains in Colorado and live out my remaining days in God's beautiful nature than die in a hospital receiving heavy and lethal doses of killer drugs and painful radiation. Who knows, I just might be cured by living under the canopy of heaven.

I heard of a story of a very successful businessman who went to the doctor complaining of experiencing spots in his eyes and ringing in his ears. This was before the era of modern medicine. The doctors did some probing and testing using what's available to them at that time and finally determined this man had a terminal illness and they gave him six months to live. The man went home and told his wife what the doctors had told him. They both informed their children. They all decided the family needed a change so they scheduled a world tour, a vacation they all needed and especially the dad. In just a few short weeks, the father remarked to his wife he had never felt better in his life.

While in France, he told his wife, "I've always wanted to have a Taylor-made suit."

His wife said, "Then have one Taylor-made."

They all agreed, after all their father and husband was going to be dead in six months. He entered the store and they did the usual measurements for a suit and tie. They got to the shirt and measured for his neck size and the Taylor said, "Your neck size is 16."

The businessman responded "No, it is 15 and a half."

The Taylor measured again and said, "It is 16, Sir."

Again, the businessman said, "I have always worn a 15 and half collar size."

Finally, the Taylor said, "Well, if you want ringing in your ears and see spots on your eyes, I'll make it 15 and a half."

You know we can all laugh at that story, but there is a lot of truth in it.

The old adage "Drugs don't cure" still holds true today. Drugs suppress the symptoms of the disease but they do not cure the disease. Most diseases are brought on by our lifestyles. As hard as that is to admit to, it is true. Yesterday, I interviewed a male patient who weighed 340 pounds plus and was 5' 11" tall. If he was standing and looked down, he couldn't see his feet unless he peered way out. He had hypertension, diabetes, GERD (gastroesophageal reflux disease), and experienced SOB (shortness of breath) because (and he said) "I am so fat." Those were his words. One good thing, he quit smoking three years ago. He was on a long list of medications, more than ten. He was scheduled for an upper and lower endoscopy. At this point in his life, medications were not controlling his GERDS, and so the doctor wanted to look into his esophagus, stomach, and small intestine for ulcers. He said he was addicted to soda pop and after further inquiry, I discovered he drank two liters of coke a day. When the surgeon was doing the upper endoscopy, someone in the surgery suite ask if the inflammation we were looking at in his esophagus and stomach could be at least partly attributable to his mega consummation of coke. The surgeon responded with, "Well, the Coca-Cola company would demand a study showing the connection." It doesn't take a rocket scientist to understand if Coca-Cola can remove rust from a nail made out of steel, it surely can inflame and eat the tender lining of your insides to pieces. This poor man had inflammation and ulcers and a serious case of GERDS for which drugs were not curing but only masking or suppressing his symptoms. This man was sick, felt and looked miserable, and was going to all the wrong places for help. He is only forty-eight years old.

I want to encourage everyone who is reading this book that you, too, can overcome type 2 diabetes by making some simple lifestyle changes. When you make these changes, you are going to have more money, more energy, less weight, feel better when you awaken in the morning, feel better when you go to bed and your sex life is going to be better.

Chapter Seven: GERD (gastroesophageal reflux disease) Got Reflux? Acidic Foods Aren't the Problem

---

Your stomach is supposed to be acidic! Acid helps to break down foods. People who take acid-blocking medications have a much higher risk of food poisoning.

– Henry S. Lodge, M.D.

Find more

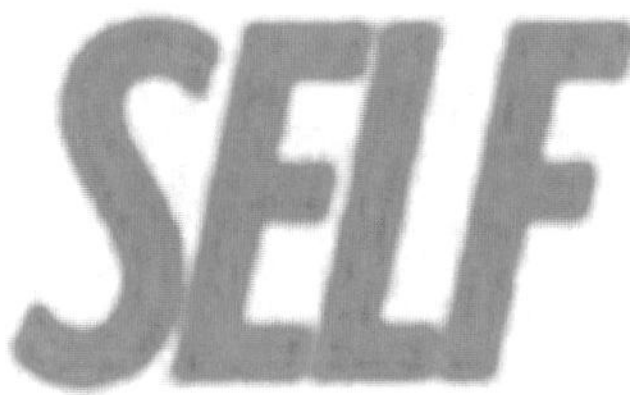

Q. I am interested in identifying foods that would be bad for someone with acid-reflux related conditions like GERD and Barrett's Esophagus. Is there something on NutritionData.com that would tell me if a food is acidic and should be avoided?

A: Nutrition Data doesn't show the acidity (pH) of foods. However, acidic foods are not what causes GERD (reflux) or heartburn.

The burning sensation and other symptoms of reflux occur when stomach acid backs up into the esophagus. Your stomach is supposed to be acidic! Acid helps to break down foods (especially proteins) for digestion and also has the important job of killing any pathogenic micro-organisms your food might contain. In fact:

People who take acid-blocking medications have a much higher risk of food poisoning.

Anyway, this acid doesn't come from foods you eat. It's produced by cells in the stomach. And as long as it stays in your stomach, there's no problem because the cells lining the stomach are specially designed to withstand the corrosive effects of stomach acid.

The lining of the esophagus is much more delicate, however. Normally, a tight ring of muscle called the lower esophageal sphincter, or LES, keeps things moving one way. Food is allowed to pass through the LES into the stomach but acid is prevented from moving up into the esophagus. If the LES fails to close tightly enough, that's when problems occur.

Pharmaceutical therapies for GERD aim to reduce the amount of acid in your stomach so that when it seeps through the LES to the esophagus it doesn't do as much damage. But reducing stomach acid has other consequences. Reducing stomach acid also impairs your ability to digest your food and absorb nutrients. For example:

People taking acid-suppressing drugs absorb less calcium and have an increased risk of bone fractures.

So the real question you want to ask isn't "Which foods are acidic?" or even "How can I reduce the amount of acid in my stomach?" but "How can I keep my stomach acid in my stomach where it belongs?"

Try these natural steps to relieve reflux:

1. Avoid clothing that's very tight around your middle. Tight waistbands or belts can squeeze the stomach, forcing the contents up against the LES.

2. Avoid overfilling your stomach. Large meals also put pressure on the LES.
3. Don't lie down after eating. Let gravity help keep stomach contents where they belong.
4. Maintain a healthy body weight. Excess abdominal fat can put pressure on the stomach contents and cause reflux.

Foods that aggravate reflux

People with reflux are often advised to avoid coffee, tomatoes, and citrus juice. But it's not because these foods are acidic. Rather, it's because they tend to relax the LES. If you suffer from reflux, you also may want to avoid peppermint, caffeinated beverages, alcohol, and tobacco, all of which also tend to relax the LES.

In my experience, these steps can frequently resolve chronic reflux. If you've had reflux for a long time and your esophagus is showing signs of damage, your doctor may want you to take an acid-suppressing drug to allow the damage to heal. But, in my opinion, acid-suppression should be a short-term intervention, not a permanent solution.

In its early stages, this is a disease that can be treated and never return by simple lifestyle changes. But again, the drug cartels don't want anyone cured from this disease. They want you to be on one or more of their drugs for the rest of your life; and they keep coming up with new drugs to treat GERDS because these drugs don't cure; they only suppress the symptoms of a deeper underlying pathology.

Just yesterday, I talked with a patient who was in his thirties and needed to have an abscess opened and drained in his right groin. It was a case that needed to be done ASAP, but he had eaten at 8:00 A.M. and it was only 2:00 P.M. and I would prefer to have eight hours from the last time a patient has eaten to the time of surgery. If you administer general anesthesia too soon after a person has eaten, that food may reflux back from the stomach into the esophagus and get into the lungs and that can spell disaster. After explaining his options or anesthesia choices, he chose to have a spinal with some sedation; I asked him, "What did you eat for breakfast at 8?" He said he ate at Hardee's where he said he eats every morning and he had biscuits and gravy and meat. I asked him, "Do you ever eat any fruit with your breakfast?" and he said, "No." He was already suffering from reflux.

He said he snacks throughout the day and eats an all-American dinner after work of meat and potatoes. Fast food eating will help send you to the grave quicker than anything I know of.

Our stomachs need rest in between meals just like every organ in our body needs rest. Even our heart muscle gets rest with every beat it makes to supply fresh, nourishing, clean blood to every cell in our bodies.

This is one of the reasons caffeinated drinks like soda pop and coffee and tea and tobacco are so damaging to our hearts. They increase our blood pressure which makes our heart muscle pump harder and increase our heart rate which takes away the time the heart muscle should be resting between each beat. Chocolate has similar effects that caffeine and nicotine have because it contains *theobromine*. What is theobromine? Theobromine, also known as *xantheuse* is a bitter alkaloid of the cacao plant, found in chocolate.

The primary *methylxanthine* in chocolate is theobromine, a molecule similar to caffeine and *theophylline*.

Chocolate is made from the cocoa bean, which is a natural source of theobromine.

I found the following information on *theobromine* from the Wikipedia.

"The amount of theobromine found in chocolate is small enough that chocolate can, in general, be safely consumed by humans. However, theobromine poisoning may result from the chronic or acute consumption of large quantities, especially in the elderly.[31]

While theobromine and caffeine are similar in that they are related alkaloids, theobromine is weaker in both its inhibition of cyclic nucleotide *phosphodiesterases* and its antagonism of adenosine receptors.[32] Therefore, theobromine has a lesser impact on human central nervous system than caffeine. However, theobromine stimulates the heart to a greater degree.[33] While theobromine is not as addictive, it has been cited as possibly causing addiction to chocolate.[34] Theobromine has also been identified as one of the compounds contributing to chocolate's reputed role as an aphrodisiac."[35]

Is it any wonder then after years of abuse the heart muscle just collapses under the consumption of coffee, caffeinated sodas and chocolate, and lack of rest and exercise; and then we wonder why we experience chest pain, a heart attack, or in some cases, sudden death. Okay, you wouldn't know if you experienced sudden death but families left behind surely do.

We must give nature time to recover because with wrong lifestyle, nature is growing weaker and is less capable of recovering from years of abuse. We have an incredible body and mind; when it was first created, it was meant to last for eternity and never give out.

If you are determined to persevere and overcome and make changes in your lifestyle, abused nature will soon again rally, and perform her work wisely and well without all the stimulants you may be presently ingesting. At the end of the day after consuming so many stimulants, your body is just exhausted and you fall prostrate in the evening with no energy left for yourself, your children, or your wife.

This wrung out feeling at the end of the day may be overcome if you get away from junk eating and stimulating drinks. When your blood pressure and heart rate go up each by ten points and basically remain there all day, how do you think you are going to feel? Those increases in blood pressure and heart rate should be increased without drugs as when we exercise and work outside in our yards and when we play with the children or whatever we happen to be doing. Then it is natural and no damage will be done if it is not done in excess.

Balance is the key in everything you do—keep the right perspective.

The next few paragraphs I got from a web site advertising Nexium, a drug promoted to treat GERDS. What is interesting is this site mentions three treatments, none of which include lifestyle changes. They do mention at the end of this advertisement that if a change in diet hasn't helped and heartburn persists for more than two or more days a week, then Nexium is the treatment for you. They also say, "Nexium is prescribed to treat the symptoms of acid reflux disease."

They don't say anything about getting at the heart of your problem, because they know if you implement some simple life style changes, you won't need their drugs.

It goes on: "When you have heartburn, there are many acid reflux treatments you can get over the counter (without a doctor's prescription). And while these may give you temporary heartburn relief, they may not be the best option for you (the drug cartels make more money on prescription drugs). If you're taking antacids more than twice a week, it could mean that the problem isn't just heartburn, but may be a more serious condition—acid reflux disease. If you think you may have acid reflux disease, talk to your doctor about the best acid reflux treatment option for you.

Three types of treatments include:

1. Antacids:
   Antacids work by neutralizing stomach acid. They can provide fast relief from occasional heartburn, but the relief is usually short-term.
2. H2 blockers:
   H2 blockers reduce acid production in the stomach by blocking a signal that leads to acid secretion. They can help heal possible damage to the esophagus that may be caused by acid reflux disease.
3. Proton pump inhibitors (PPIs)
   Proton pump inhibitors—like NEXIUM—are proven to be the most effective treatments for acid reflux disease. They work by turning off some of the "acid pumps" in the stomach's acid-producing cells. Most PPIs are available only with a doctor's prescription. PPIs can both relieve heartburn pain and heal possible damage to the esophagus that may be caused over time by acid reflux disease.

NEXIUM is prescribed to treat the symptoms of acid reflux disease, which typically include persistent heartburn on two or more days per week, despite treatment and change of diet."

In this above advertisement for nexium it says this drug works by "turning off some of the 'acid pumps' in the stomachs acid producing cells."

But guess what, there is a reason why the stomach has acid producing cells. It didn't come just by chance that our stomach has acid producing cells. The human body and mind are so closely connected they function as one unit. In other words, what affects one affects the other. Does that sound even oddly familiar, something you may have heard from your grandmother? One of my favorite authors writing on health over a hundred years ago wrote this:

"The sympathy which exists between the mind and the body is very great. When one is affected, the other responds" (MH pp. 230).

Wow! How simple is that? Yes, that's right. It's something our grandparents knew. When the mind is depressed, the body will soon experience weakness and sometimes disease will follow if the depression isn't addressed. That is why exercise is so important. When we hurt ourselves or contract a cold, a flu, or some kind of disease, the right attitude in the mind can bring healing to the mind. A healthy body and a healthy mind are in sync; if the body and mind are not in sync, you will see or experience from a few to an untold number of symptoms.

The reason over the counter medications like antacids are sold without a prescription and in just about every food store is they are not really that effective or dangerous. It is like getting ready for the Fourth of July celebration in the United States of America. We used to be able to buy pretty powerful fireworks—like cherry bombs—and some of you reading this know what I'm talking about; but now the fireworks you are able to purchase are fairly benign. And the drug cartels are making billions of dollars from the sale of over the counter medications. Most of these drugs are sold because people are seeking a quick fix to their ailing health. They don't want to make any lifestyle changes; changes that are so simple, changes that don't cost anything; changes that are free.

Most people just want a quick fix because they feel they can't take time to make lifestyle changes.

With the new Obama healthcare reform bill, many of the drugs people take for granted that they could take almost daily may soon disappear. Why? Because as a nation, we are almost bankrupt.

Pharmaceutical companies will stop making a drug if they see their revenue for that drug waning. In defense of pharmaceutical companies, they spend millions in research to even get a drug approved by the FDA, then they must spend millions more to advertise the new medication. But when the time elapses for their exclusive rights to produce a certain drug expires, then any other drug company can also produce the same drug under a generic name; therefore, their profit margin many times goes out the window.

I have witnessed this a few times in my career where we have been administering a particular medication, say, for post-op nausea and vomiting and it has been working well and then one day our hospital pharmacists informs us that medication will no longer be available. Why? Well I have heard a variety of reasons, but most of the time it will come down to money; because when other pharmaceutical companies begin making generic brands of the same drug and its effects are clearly the same or sometimes better than the parent drug, then the parent drug companies' profits are going to fall sharply.

Now if you are a businessperson, you are probably thinking, *That's how you run a business*. I would agree with you on that principle. You must make a profit on what you are selling or you cannot continue to manufacture that product; but I thought from all the millions of dollars spent on advertising about how these companies care to help you that they would surely continue to produce a drug with a lower profit margin, especially after making millions or even billions on some drugs over a period of several years.

Just last week I was taking a history from a patient who was scheduled for a hysterectomy. She was positive for hypertension and GERD. I asked what medications she was taking to control the symptoms associated with her hypertension and GERD. She responded, "I'm not." I asked "Why?" She said, "I can't afford to buy them." I hear this all the time. "I can't afford to buy the medications I need." I am especially concerned with the aging population who are on a fixed income that cannot afford to purchase the drugs they have been on for years, and who now are dependent on the daily fix of drugs. You see, this is what the drug cartels want; they want you dependent upon them to provide you with drugs that you have actually become addicted to. They don't care two cents about your well-being. They actually don't want you to get cured, because if the drug alone could cure you of your disease, you would no longer need to buy their drugs. They are just like blood succors. It kind of sounds much like big government, doesn't it? Big government wants you to be dependent upon them; and yes, at least for now, the drug cartels (pharmaceutical companies) are in the pockets of big government.

Now, you may not be able to stop some of the things that will ensue big government; but as for your health, there is a lot you can do. You can take back control of your body and mind. This is what medications that you don't need long term do. They control you—and that is when medications (something that aides in healing) become drugs (something that harms you) and you become addicted and dependent upon the pharmaceutical companies (drug cartels).

Some of these drugs cost hundreds of dollars a month. This is one of the reasons insurance rates have skyrocketed. Everyone wants the best insurance plan. They want an insurance coverage that covers all their medication costs. Nobody wants to pay a dime out of one's own pockets. The sad thing about all of this is that if you would make some simple lifestyle changes, you wouldn't need all those drugs—and that, my dear friend, means more money in your pocket.

Do you want to be healthier and happier and have more money to spend to enjoy life to the fullest? Yes, I'm sure you do, and most people do. Well then, as far as possible get off medications that have become drugs and that you are dependent upon or that you are addicted to.

Don't ever stop taking medications that you have been on without first consulting a physician, because you may experience some very severe rebound symptoms or side effects. This is particularly true with blood pressure and depression or bipolar medications. Again, this is exactly what the drug cartels want. There is no freedom like freedom from the bondage of drugs. Ask any recovering addict. I'll touch on this later, but the single most abused drug used today is alcohol. Yes, alcohol is a drug.

Negative intrathoracic pressure (ITP) and positive elevation of intra-gastric and intra-abdominal pressures (IGP and IAP) tend to promote reflux. Simply stated, when you have more pressure in your stomach than you have in your esophagus or when the pressure in your stomach exceeds the pressure in your esophagus, the cardiac sphincter (the barrier between the stomach and the esophagus) opens, and you will experience the unpleasant taste of food coming back up your esophagus.

That unpleasant taste usually returns because acid is refluxing or leaking back into the esophagus and traveling up into your oral pharynx, mouth, sinuses, and down into your lungs, causing untold damage to those areas of your body.

Every time I take a history from a patient going to surgery, the same patient I will be giving a general anesthetic to, I always ask him or her for any history of gastric or acid reflux.

Just the other day, I was taking a history from a twenty-eight-year-old female scheduled for a upper (EGD) and lower (colonoscopy). I ask her what her eating habits or schedule was for each day. Basically, I wanted to know what her lifestyle was, because lifestyle is much more than eating and drinking, as we will see later on in this book. She looked as if she was twenty years older than what her birth date revealed. She was a two-pack a day smoker, and she looked as if she hadn't slept in the last week. Her facial cheeks were sunken, which told me she had poor tissue turgor and muscle wasting.

She told me she never ate breakfast, but she always started her day with a diet cola and of course, a cigarette. On her break at work, she would have another diet cola. She did not eat lunch, but she always had another diet cola. She would usually have some type of meat, usually a fish sandwich and chips for dinner, and of course another diet cola. She said she never eats fruits or vegetables and rarely drinks water. Then I asked how many diet colas she drinks each day. She said she consumed from between nine and eleven diet colas and smoked two packs of cigarettes every day.

I just interviewed a patient a few days ago with an interesting story and I asked her if I could place it in my book and she readily agreed. She was about thirty-seven years of age; when I asked her if she has any urinary history, she immediately said, "Not now." She said for seven years she experienced frequent urinary tract infections, UTI's. Then while seeing a doctor over in North Carolina about her UTI's, he asked her about how many soft drinks she was consuming a day. She was drinking twenty-four cans of soda pop a day—Coca Cola, Doctor Pepper, and Mountain Dew. He advised her to cut out soda pop and she would not have UTI's. Three years ago, she quit drinking all soda pops "cold turkey," and has been free of UTI's for the past three years—but the manufacturers of soft drinks are not going to tell you the harmful effects of their products.

I've heard similar stories over twenty-seven years of taking histories from patients going to surgery. But before me was a twenty-eight-year old female who looked like death warmed over. My heart went out to her as it does to everyone I see living a lifestyle of multiple addictions. Everybody when he or she is born has some type of addictive behavior, although it may never become a problem or issue for some. There are two main reasons for this: 1. the lifestyle given by parents or the lifestyle ultimately chosen for themselves, and 2. heredity.

The distressing and appalling thing about this whole scenario with this twenty-eight year old lady is she was now showing symptoms caused almost solely by her lifestyle. No one needed to tell her she needed to stop smoking and quit drinking diet colas, but we all did—from her doctor, to her nurse, and to myself, who would administer her anesthesia. She would now undergo an upper endoscopy called an EGD and a lower endoscopy called a colonoscopy.

Both of these procedures have their own inherent risks. Any time you administer anesthesia, a patient is placed at risk. Certainly, when you are passing a scope about five feet long up the rectum and traverse the large intestine to the end of the small intestine where the appendix is located, there are increased risks. Some endoscopists are not satisfied until they have at least entered the small intestine. I have had a couple of patients ask me—after they have been sedated and I'm standing at their head and just before they get sedated to where they're not talking—"So what is your job during my colonoscopy?"

Sometimes, after I have established a good rapport, I would respond, "I let your doctor know when the scope is coming out of your mouth," but really, the patients know I'm kidding. They laugh and they actually take less anesthesia because "Laughter is the best medicine."

When I was in Colorado, I had a patient say to me, "Hey, Doc, if you don't find my head up there, tell my wife, because she's been telling me for twenty-five years my head is up my ___."

What can happen during this procedure? You can end up with a ruptured colon from the scope perforating through the wall of the large intestine. If that happens, the patient now has free air inside the abdominal cavity and fecal material can now pass into a sterile area. At this point, it is kind of like having a ruptured appendix. Immediate surgery is now required and depending on the health status of the patient, he or she may do well, or experience an extended stay in the hospital—or in the worse-case scenario, ultimately die.

Do I recommend a colonoscopy at times? Absolutely! For the health insurance I have for my family, a colonoscopy does not cost me a dime because it is considered a preventive treatment. I have administered anesthesia for literally thousands of colonoscopies and can count on one hand the number of perforating colons we had to take to surgery and repair a ruptured colon. Have I had a colonoscopy? Yes. When I was fifty-two years old, I was experiencing some rectal bleeding.

The report came back negative. They didn't find any polyps. The doctor said I just had some internal hemorrhoids that were causing the bleeding.

Although my dad lived to be eighty-three and my mother lived to be eighty-nine, neither one had ever had an upper or lower endoscopy. But they grew up in a different age and lived a very good lifestyle. They were both vegetarians and I can't remember a time they ever ate out. Right now, I have taken a hiatus on eating out at any kind of restaurant. By avoiding restaurants and eating at home more, or when you're traveling, buy some finger foods like nuts, dried or fresh fruits and fresh veggies; you will escape or elude some potentially dangerous health problems like obesity, diabetes, hypertension, GERDS and the list goes on. And you guessed right: These all may be prevented by a simple change in lifestyle. Isn't that great!

There are many advertisements out there, especially on the internet, about cleansing your colon; for the most part, these advertisements are full of misinformation at the least and are bordering on medical malpractice at the worst.

Q: Do colon detox products work, and are they safe?

A: No, and they can be dangerous, says Richard Harkness, a consultant pharmacist and author of five books on evidence-based natural medicine. "Colon cleansing" procedures are based on the faulty theory that fecal matter and toxins—such as parasites, pesticides, or chemicals—accumulate and stick to the colon wall, causing assorted ailments. In fact, fecal matter does not cling to the colon wall, and experts have found no evidence that toxins build up there."

The best way to cleanse the colon is to begin by fasting from eating anything but fresh fruits and drinking eight to ten eight-ounce glasses of water a day. Stay on this regimen for one week and you will notice an incredible change. At the end of the week for one day, drink only water eight to twelve eight-ounce glasses.

After this, you can go back to eating two or three meals a day; but eat sparingly for the next three days because your stomach has shrunk a little. You will probably notice you have lost a little weight and you may find your pants don't fit as tightly as before. This is all good; and guess what, your colon is clean and it didn't cost you a dime. Furthermore, you didn't place the electrolytes in your body out of balance, which can be very dangerous physiologically.

Colon cleansing is a money-making scam and like the latest fad diet, almost everybody from "No-Where's-Ville" is trying to make a quick and easy buck at your financial and physical well-being.

Just add plenty of fresh fruit and fresh vegetables to your diet every day and your colon will stay as clean as it was designed to.

That's why I am writing this book; I want to give you the encouragement and the know-how to live a happy and full life. It is so rewarding to wake up each day in good health, full of energy, and to know you have taken back control of your life. I love living life to the fullest. How about you?

If you are suffering from acid reflux, then follow these simple steps and within thirty days you will not have acid reflux. Here are the steps:

1. Stop drinking caffeinated drinks, cut out coffee, don't drink alcohol, and stop eating chocolate. Drinking these things impairs the LES (lower esophageal sphincter), the door between your stomach and esophagus that keeps food and acid from backing up into your esophagus from your stomach.
2. Stop eating between meals. Your stomach needs five hours between meals for full recovery from the last ingestion of food.
3. Eat more sparingly at each meal and take at least twenty minutes to eat. It takes about twenty minutes for your stomach to receive a signal from your brain that you are full. This will keep you from gorging yourself. Chew your food thoroughly and don't drink anything with your meals, not even water.

After you eat, don't lie down and if you are able to, take a little walk. Remember, when the pressure in your stomach exceeds the pressure in your esophagus, you will experience acid reflux—it's as simple as that; or if you continue to drink coffee and caffeinated drinks and consume alcohol and use chocolate, you will finally and permanently damage your LES and that little door (or your LES) between your stomach and your esophagus will remain partially open permanently. And, finally, have at least five hours from your last meal until the time you go to bed.

Keep in mind that if you don't change your lifestyle to eliminate or at least bring under control acid reflux, you will begin to experience things like gastritis, esophagitis, rhinitis, and bronchitis and if you have acid reflux long enough, you may end up with some form of cancer like esophageal cancer.

You might be already saying to yourself this is too complicated, but really—it's not. After just thirty days of implementing and implanting these simple lifestyle changes, they will become part of your everyday lifestyle and the rewards will be incredible.

Chapter Eight: Obesity

"Metabolic Syndrome" is a cluster of health risk factors. These include having a fat stomach, high cholesterol, high blood pressure, and high blood sugar. These problems affect over fourteen million Americans and the cost for treatment is about $1,700.00 a year. That makes this a twenty-seven trillion dollar problem—just in the United States. How many of these factors do you have?

Some doctors have said that people with cancer are much "better" patients than those who have metabolic syndrome, because cancer patients take the doctor's advice seriously, are grateful for the advice, and follow the advice. Metabolic syndrome patients ignore the doctor's advice and are generally annoyed to get the advice year after year. Why would these patients ignore this advice? Cancer patients are afraid they will die and so they view the doctor's advice as a lifeline. On the other hand, "those with metabolic syndrome slowly progress to diabetes and heart disease. Those patients think there is no rush to reform." (*Adult Sabbath School Lesson Study Outlines*).

Obesity is classified according to the body mass index or BMI expressed in Weight kilograms divided by height in meters squared or BMI = wt kg ÷ by ht m2.

Following are two examples of the calculation of BMI.

Woman 5 feet 4 inches tall weighing 126 pounds:
126 lbs ÷ 2.2kg/lb = 57 kg
5ft 4 in or 64 in x 2.54 cm/in=1.63 m
1.63 squared (1.63 x 1.63) = 2.66
BMI = 57 ÷ 2.66 = 21.4

Woman 5 feet 4 inches tall weighing 220 pounds:
220 lbs ÷ 2.2 kg/lb = 100 kg
5ft 4 in or 64 in x 2.54 cm/in = 1.63m
1.63squared = 2.66
BMI = 100 ÷ 2.66 = 37.6

Classification of Obesity

BMI(kg/m2)	Category
< 18	Underweight
19-24	Normal weight
25-59	Overweight
30-39	Obese
35	Morbidly obese if comorbid factors exist
40	Morbidly obese
50	Super obese

One quick and easier method—but not quite as accurate—for measuring obesity is to take your height in inches where both sexes at 60 inches or 5 feet would equal 100 pounds. Now, for every inch in addition to 60 you add 6 pounds for men and 5 pounds for women; then take into account bone size. For small bone size, deduct 5-10 percent and for large bone size, add 5-10 percent. So if you are a male and are 6 feet tall, that equals 72 inches; therefore 60 inches would equal 100 pounds and add 72 pounds for 12 inches multiplied by 6 pounds per inch and you should weigh 172 pounds if your bone size is average and you are a male. If your bone size is large, add 5-10 percent or 8-17 pounds. If your bone size is small, then deduct 5-10 percent or 8-17 pounds.

My weight stays at about 160 pounds. I am 5'10" tall and have average bone size; therefore, with this rough but easy calculation, I should weigh about 160 pounds. Fortunately, for now, my weight is between 158 lbs-162 lbs, based upon this calculation formula.

If you look at other countries, people in North America are on the average larger or heavier. Hans Diehl, DrHSc, MPH, and Aileen Ludington, MD, in their introduction to the little pamphlet entitled "Reversing Obesity" aptly portray problems with obesity in North America:

Obesity is one of our leading public health problems. So severe is this disease that 36 million people are at serious medical risk.

Being overweight shortens life. It also lays the foundation for nearly every degenerative disease except osteoporosis. Obese people are three times more likely to have heart disease, four times more likely to suffer from high blood pressure, five times more likely to develop diabetes and elevated blood cholesterols, and six times more likely to have gallbladder disease. They also develop more cancer of the colon, rectum, prostate, breast, cervix, uterus and ovaries, and suffer more osteoarthritis and low back pain. Overweight people are like ticking bombs waiting for one or more of these diseases to explode in their lives.

In addition, extra weight affects self-image. In today's appearance-oriented society, it can be a great psychological burden.

What's needed is a dietary lifestyle that maintains health, increases energy, lowers the risk of disease, reduces food bills, and allows people to eat as much as they want and still lose weight without feeling hungry.

The other day, my wife prepared a total vegan supper. She had burritos stuffed full of brown rice, different vegetables, including spinach. I then added on the outside of the burrito diced up lettuce, tomatoes, onions, and avocadoes. It was delicious; but the amazing thing is you didn't feel stuffed when you were done eating. Also, you could eat as much as you desired and still lose weight. That is what Hans Diehl and Aileen Ludington were writing about when they wrote, "People can eat as much as they want and still lose weight without feeling hungry."

What gives you that stuffed feeling are all those empty calories in foods and drinks and all the fat and salt and preservatives added to our foods. It's no wonder people feel bloated after eating a large meal.

And it's not just what you're eating but how and when you're eating. Millions of Americans are mostly meat and potato consumers, usually eaten late in the evening. Only in the last few years has there been an attempt to get Americans to add more dietary fiber, bulk, and roughage to their diet in the form of fruits and vegetables. What does all that dietary fiber, bulk, and roughage do for our bodies? The structural part of plants and plant products that consists of carbohydrates, as cellulose and pectin, that are wholly or partially indigestible and when eaten stimulate peristalsis in the intestine. These are foods containing high amounts of such carbohydrates as whole grains, fruits, and vegetables.

When these foods are added to a meat and potato diet, they help get all that rot gut putrefying cancer producing meat out of the colon sooner. You can always tell a meat and potatoes person if you follow them after they've gone to the restroom. There is usually a foul and offensive odor. Why wouldn't there be? The meat you eat is continuing to decay and rot in your stomach and intestine. If you have meat in your home, do you leave it out sitting on the counter after bringing it home from the grocery store? No, you place it into the refrigerator or freezer as soon as possible. Well, your stomach and colon is very warm compared to a freezer or refrigerator and the meat you eat is really going to start to decay quickly inside of your body.

A couple of generations ago, about sixty years, the structure of our society was much different than it is today. The industrial revolution was in full steam and running strong. If you didn't have a job, you just didn't sit back and expect the government to support you. Many people still lived on large and small farms across this great country from California to the New York islands. Freedom reigned. The cold war was on, the military was strong and terrorism as we know it today didn't exist, even Hollywood gave us good movies and programs *like I Love Lucy*, *Andy Griffith*, *My Three Sons*, and many others. If you were looking to fulfill your dreams, all you had to do was to work hard, expect much and you would be successful. We were an industrious nation. Other nations envied the United States and thousands upon thousands were moving to America in search of their dreams and many found those dreams fulfilled in America. But by and large we were active and robust, a society on the move.

About thirty years ago, I was in the office of the mayor of a little town in rural America. As I was visiting with the mayor, I noticed on the wall in his office a picture of him wearing a back brace standing in one of the manholes on one of the streets in his town. I asked him, "Why were you working with a back brace in place? Couldn't you get on workers compensation or something else so you could be off of work while your back healed?"

He responded, "There was no workers compensation programs then; besides, I couldn't have done that ethically." Wow, how times have changed. Many people are looking for ways to get on some form of government assistance or entitlement program so they don't have to work.

Now, many people in other nations do not envy America as they use to. I have talked with several people over the last couple of years who are from formerly communist regimes and they came to America to the land of dreams and opportunity and freedom, but they now see their hopes dashed and say the United States is fast approaching what they fled from—big government with little freedoms and the end to free enterprise as all Americans have come to enjoy and love.

When you take away the desire and passion for a person to work by the government promising they'll take care of you, you are removing the very foundation on which this country was founded upon—religious freedom, small government, and the very essence of our souls—INTEGRITY.

Russians were promised the government would take care of all their needs and provide everything for them but they couldn't, shouldn't, and didn't. One thing a government can never give you is integrity—it must be earned.

Most houses had front porches and in the evenings, you would actually see people sitting outside talking. Although I grew up in the country in a rural setting, I remember going into town and walking down different streets with my friends and we would pass by homes and many times people would say "hi" from their front porches, and if they knew me, they may inquire on how my parents were.

The world has changed and of course, we see that change more clearly in America than in any other place. When my daughter, Elizabeth ,was in, I believe, the ninth grade a freshman in high school, she had a home-work assignment in which she had to ask her parents some questions about how life was when they were growing up. She came to me and asked, "Dad, what did you have when you grew up?" I knew what she meant so I told her, "It is easier for me to tell you what we didn't have when I was your age. We didn't have cell phones, computers, calculators, the internet, iPods, CD's, DVD's. There were no Blockbusters to rent movies. We had one black and white television, we could only bring in three channels, and we had to wrap the rabbit ear antennas in tin foil if we wanted good reception and there was no remote control so every time we wanted to change the channel we had to get off our duff and walk over to the television and do it manually. There was no cable television or direct TV. I saw the wheels turning in her mind and she finally said, "So what did you do for fun?"

So we have moved from a very active people to a very sedentary life style. It seems as little consequence not having a remote control to change the channels on your television so that you had to get up and walk over and change channels and walk back to your seat, but you were more active. Kids and grown-ups alike sit for hours before the computer and before the television every day without virtually moving a muscle.

A nurse I worked with in Denver, Colorado, said to me one day during the Christmas season, "My husband told me to just bring home a urinal, that's all I want for Christmas, so I don't have to get up and go to the bathroom when I'm watching television." We have become a very fat, lazy, and consequently sick society.

By the time you read this book, and in particular this next article, the statistics may have already changed, but it still is applicable.

States with the Most Couch Potatoes

by Greg Bocquet
Tuesday, March 22, 2011
provided by

MAIN ST

In the earliest days of the U.S., the frontier was a tough place to live. Surely, more than one pioneer, upon reaching the rushing and roiling Mississippi River, turned to his wagon-mates and said, with a wave of his hand, "Yeah, this looks like a nice place to settle, let's call it a day."

Whatever heartiness allowed people to settle successfully in the West may have been diluted by internal migration during the past two centuries, but to get an idea of how much different states vary in their residents' fitness levels, *Main Street* looked at the Centers for Disease Control and Prevention *State Indicator Report on Physical Activity, 2010*.

The report addresses a number of characteristics related to fitness—both behavioral indicators (how often you exercise) and environmental (how many parks and playgrounds there are in the area, etc.)—but boils down the principal ranking to the "proportion of adults in the state who achieve at least 150 minutes a week of moderate-intensity aerobic physical activity or 75 minutes a week of vigorous-intensity aerobic physical activity or an equivalent combination of moderate- and vigorous-intensity aerobic activity."

Here we look at the ten states at the bottom of that list, so that the couch potatoes can go about addressing the problem.

As the CDC says, "When state officials, health professionals, nonprofit organizations, urban planners, parks and recreation representatives, school staff, transportation officials, and community members work together, their efforts can increase the number of Americans who live healthier lives by creating communities that support and encourage physical activity."

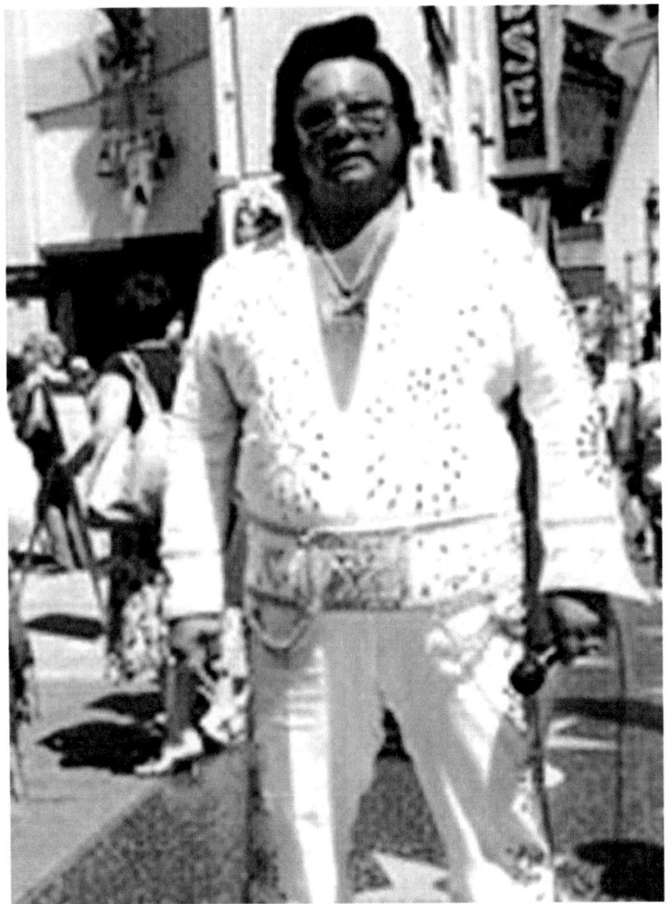

©cardigan/flickr

1. Tennessee

Physically active adults: 51.8 percent

Taking the top spot as the laziest state in the union is Tennessee, where just more than half—51.8 percent—of the adult population report at least two and a half hours of physical activity per week. The state also played host to one of the most notorious expanding waistlines in pop culture, as *Elvis Presley spent his last years in Memphis* in a spiral of drug abuse, overeating, and, yes, general laziness. The only ray of sunshine for energetic Tennesseans who would rather see their state off this list altogether, the CDC found that 24.3 percent of the state's high school students report moderate physical activity, a comforting statistic in light of the 17.1 percent national average.

2. Louisiana

Physically active adults: 56 percent

In a state known for decadent beignets and the "po boy," a foot-long submarine sandwich slathered in gravy and, sometimes, tartar sauce, only 56 percent of adults report moderate to vigorous physical activity with any kind of regularity. While there is no data in the CDC report for physical activity among high school students, one detail stands out as a possible indicator of the future fitness of Louisianans: only 35.5 percent of the state's youth have parks, community centers, and sidewalks in the neighborhood, far below the national average of 50 percent.

3. Mississippi

Physically active adults: 57.2 percent

Kicking off the top three is Mississippi, home to the purported descendants of some of the aforementioned lazy pioneers. Indeed, the state ranks number one for the proportion of its adults who report "no leisure-time physical activity" at 32.4 percent. That's almost a third of adults who are not embarrassed to report to the CDC that they get basically no regular physical exercise. It also ranks number one for the prevalence of obesity, as a 2009 CDC report registered *34.4 percent of Mississippi's population as obese*, the highest of any state.

4. Kentucky

Physically active adults: 57.9 percent

Kentucky, whether it wants to or not, is known throughout the world for its fried chicken recipe popularized by Col. Sanders. While deep-fried anything is delicious, it should really be enjoyed with a side dish of vigorous exercise. Unfortunately for most Kentuckians, there doesn't seem to be as many opportunities to get that exercise as there should be: The CDC reports that only 10.1 percent of census blocks have a park, half the national average of 20.3 percent.

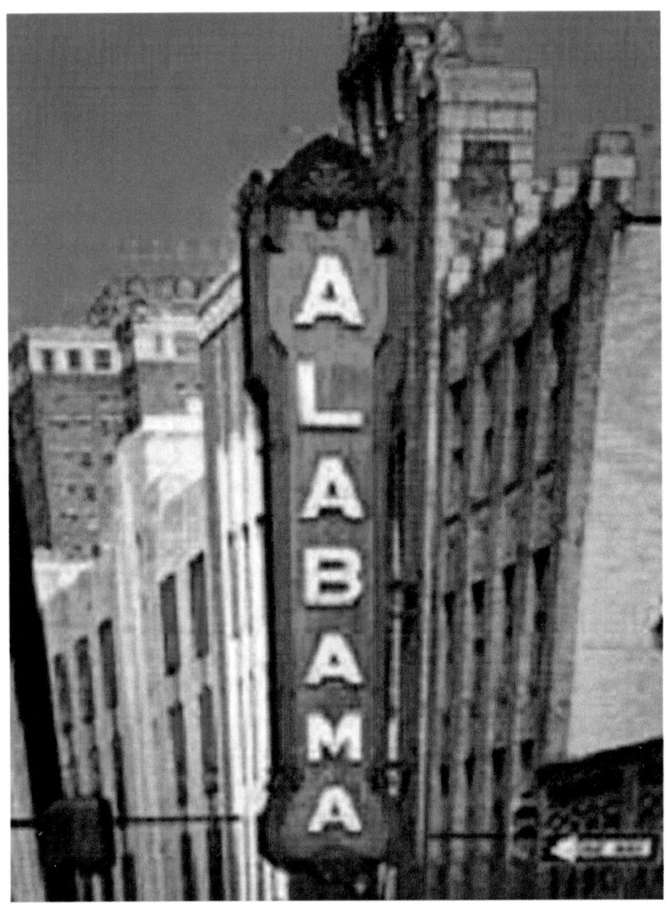

5. Alabama

Physically active adults: 59 percent

The first state on our list to fall below 60 percent of adults who exercise is Alabama, a state that was also in the top ten for obesity in 2009, with fully *31 percent of the population defined as obese*. The numbers aren't surprising when considering a few other characteristics that the CDC highlighted in its report: Alabama does not require or recommend elementary schools to provide scheduled recess, its child care centers don't specify moderate or vigorous physical activity, and the state doesn't support urban design, land use, and transportation policies that promote physical activity. These facts don't bode well for the future fitness of the state, and the lack of data on high school students suggests officials take a closer look at the "heart of Dixie."

6. North Carolina

Physically active adults: 60.9 percent

North Carolina is an interesting state in terms of its characteristics of physical activity. At number six, not even 61 percent of North Carolinian adults report much exercise, but in other ways, the state seems to be addressing the problem. Fewer adults report no physical activity than the national average (24.5 percent as opposed to 25.4 percent of American adults in general), and young people are quite active, with 24.5 percent of high school students reporting moderate physical activity compared to the 17.1 percent for the nation as a whole.

"Ain't Never Gonna Change" is the Southern motto.

Just two generations ago we were a much more agrarian or pastoral people, simple and undignified living out the American dream of owning our own house and some land whether it was a large or small piece; we would someday own it and big government couldn't take it away from us. There were little country schools through-out our nation where children walked or rode their bikes to and from school every day. My mother was born at home in 1913 in the same farm house that her father was born in, and in the house that her fathers' father her grandfather built from the trees from his own property cut by his own sawmill. When I was a young lad, I would play near the saw mill because at that time the trees had all grown up around it; I remember dreaming of how it might have been when the saw mill was in full operation.

Now, you want to talk about active, but back then, there was no time to sit down and stare at a computer or television for hours every day. Everyone had to pitch in and do his or her part. Work ethics have all but been lost in our society, replaced by entitlement programs and situation ethics where there is no right or wrong. Work brings dignity to ourselves and a feeling of accomplishment and working together as a family brings love and joy to the home. If we could somehow return to, at least in part, of how our grandparents and great grandparents lived, we would be happier, healthier, and wealthier, and the divorce rate would plummet, ADHD would all but disappear and many lifestyle diseases would become non-existent. Are there any of these things that you wouldn't desire?

Years ago when my wife was a nurse for three OBGYN doctors, one day one of the doctors, Doctor Knecht, said to her, "Where did you get such good work ethics?" Her mother and father were hard workers, and that was passed down to my wife. Her grandparents were hard workers; so my wife had good work ethics in her genes—it was hereditary. You can't take a course in work ethics and expect your children to be excited about working. They have to grow up in a culture where it is just part of their lifestyle.

I'm writing this book from a small one-bedroom apartment in a six-unit apartment complex and so we have some small children running around here. Just yesterday morning before leaving for the hospital to work, I took some trash over to the dumpster and passed by two young ladies and a little boy about two years of age. What caught my eye was the little boy wasn't walking or riding a tricycle, he was riding around in a little motorized four-wheeler.

We all have to change our mindset on how we think. We need to think about how I can get more exercise in with a slower pace in life.

But never forget today is tomorrow for the rest of your life. That means whatever decisions you make today can and will affect you for the rest of your life and the sooner all of us change our lifestyles the sooner we will be changing the outcome of our lives for tomorrow.

Do I want to get rid of all our modern technology? No, but I would like us to use them as tools and not let them become crutches, that if we found ourselves without them, that we couldn't survive. Television and computers have stifled and almost extinguished our imagination and creativity, especially in young people.

Ask yourself at the end of the day, "Did I have more time for meditation, relaxation, and time to spend with my wife and kids, because of my cell phone, iPods, and computers?" If you answered yes to that, modern technology is a blessing to you; but if your answer is no, then modern technology has become a curse to you. You make the call—because it is ultimately your call.

If you really want to see your creativity and imagination return, take a one-week break from all things technological like television, computers, cell phones, iPods, and go camping, take a long needed vacation, or do something for somebody else.

Today you hear a lot of talk about going green and the government is passing every kind of rule and regulation to enforce their green agenda. Former Vice-President Al Gore has made millions of dollars pushing the green agenda while driving gas-guzzling SUV's and not implanting or implementing many of the things he preaches and writes about.

Just yesterday, I received an email from a good friend who puts in proper perspective the hoax of going green.

> *Old memories...which we tend to 'forget' with all the 'modern' inventions...we really were much 'greener' back when......lol*

In the line at the store, the cashier told the older woman that she should bring her own grocery bag because plastic bags weren't good for the environment.

The woman apologized to him and explained, "We didn't have the green thing back in my day."

The clerk responded, "That's our problem today. The former generation did not care enough to save our environment." He was right, that generation didn't have the green thing in its day.

Back then, they returned their milk bottles, soda bottles, and beer bottles to the store. The store sent them back to the plant to be washed and sterilized and refilled, so it could use the same bottles over and over. So they really were recycled.

But they didn't have the green thing back in that customer's day.

In her day, they walked up stairs, because they didn't have an escalator in every store and office building. They walked to the grocery store and didn't climb into a 300-horsepower machine every time they had to go two blocks.

But she was right. They didn't have the green thing in her day.

Back then, they washed the baby's diapers because they didn't have the throw-away kind. They dried clothes on a line, not in an energy-gobbling machine burning up 220 volts—wind and solar power really did dry the clothes.

Kids got hand-me-down clothes from their brothers or sisters, not always brand-new clothing. But that old lady is right, they didn't have the green thing back in her day.

Back then, they had one TV or radio in the house—not a TV in every room. And the TV had a small screen the size of a handkerchief, not a screen the size of the state of Montana. In the kitchen, they blended and stirred by hand because they didn't have electric machines to do everything for you.

When they packaged a fragile item to send in the mail, they used a wadded up old newspaper to cushion it, not Styrofoam or plastic bubble wrap. Back then, they didn't fire up an engine and burn gasoline just to cut the lawn. They used a push mower that ran on human power. They exercised by working so they didn't need to go to a health club to run on treadmills that operate on electricity.

But she's right, they didn't have the green thing back then. They drank from a fountain when they were thirsty instead of using a cup or a plastic bottle every time they had a drink of water.

They refilled their writing pens with ink instead of buying a new pen, and they replaced the razor blades in a razor instead of throwing away the whole razor just because the blade got dull.

But they didn't have the green thing back then. Back then, people took the streetcar or a bus and kids rode their bikes to school or rode the school bus instead of turning their moms into a twenty-four-hour taxi service.

They had one electrical outlet in a room, not an entire bank of sockets to power a dozen appliances. And they didn't need a computerized gadget to receive a signal beamed from satellites 2,000 miles out in space in order to find the nearest pizza joint.

But isn't it sad, the current generation laments how wasteful the old folks were just because they didn't have the green thing back then?

Ten Commandments to Reduce Overweight In Children:

1. Thou shalt breastfeed your baby.
2. Thou shalt not allow your child to watch television until six years old.
3. Thou shalt let your child play thirty minutes a day at your yard or playground.
4. Thou shalt not allow soft drinks in your house.
5. Thou shalt make sure your child have a full and unhurried breakfast.
6. Thou shalt encourage your child to walk to school if distance is shorter than a mile.
7. Thou shalt encourage your child to take up yoga or martial arts.
8. Thou shalt let your child join a physical education program.
9. Thou shalt enroll your child in a school that promotes good nutrition.
10. Thou shalt live in a community that supports and promotes walking, biking, and similar activities.

Leo Leonidas, MD, FAAP, Assistant Clinical Professor in Pediatrics, Tufts University School of Medicine, Boston; Attending Pediatrician

I know a lot of parents who let their children eat late in the evening and a lot of what they eat at that time is not healthy. If you are doing this or if you are encouraging your kids to eat in between meals, you are setting your children up for some real weight issues later in life; and along with weight issues come self-esteem problems and a whole list of other complications that our children do not need.

There are some very simple things you can do to lose weight:

Start an exercise program. Turn the television off, get away from your computer, get outside, and begin by walking. At first, you may not be able to walk very far, but that's okay; just take a step. There was a man who recently entered a lifestyle program and they started their residents walking early every morning. He couldn't walk more than twenty-five steps without becoming short of breath and he would have to sit and rest a spell. Well, they told him that's okay, and they encouraged him to try and go beyond the twenty-five steps the next day and he did; and within a couple of weeks he was walking four miles without becoming short of breath. They also had him on a vegetarian diet, with lots of fruits and vegetables. He was now drinking lots of water, where before he started the lifestyle program he was drinking mainly soda pops and coffee. He was now going to bed early and getting up early and eating a good breakfast. He no longer ate anything between meals.

At the hospital, I listen to mothers share with each other how busy they are going home after work and then they have to run little Johnny to soccer practice or to football practice, take Susie to cheerleading practice, or to swimming lessons, or to volleyball practice, or basketball practice or to a hundred other things that society deems necessary to raise your child.

I've got good news for you: The NAKED TRUTH is you don't have to cart your children around to every extra-curricular activity that society has offered for your little ones to grow up and become successful; because honestly, those things do not guarantee little Johnnie's or little Susie's success. As a parent, your job is not to make your child happy; it is to provide a safe environment, physically, psychologically, and spiritually; and teach them how to work and show them love and make them feel secure and—guess what—they will have integrity and they will be happy. I believe in offering my children certain things that I feel will help them grow in every way mentioned above but I'm not going to run around and involve them in everything that everyone else is in involved in, just because it happens to be popular.

A friend of mine shared with me an article I want to pass along to you. It was written by Family Psychologist John Rosemond:

Q: In a recent column, you said that parents should not be involved with their children. This isn't what we parents are being encouraged, from every direction, to do. Can you elaborate?

A: I will begin by saying, please observe my definition of "involved" in the rest of this column before you write me off.

Like most post-1960s parenting mantras, "Get involved with your kids" is accepted, not because it is common sense or has proven to be advantageous (because it hasn't), but because it has a warm and fuzzy feel to it.

For example, schools keep pushing for parental involvement in homework, claiming it results in higher achievement, yet the rise in parental participation in homework has coincided with *declines* in student achievement. There's a thin line between being involved and being interested, supportive, and encouraging. I believe it is more functional for all concerned that parents stay, for the most part, on the interested and supportive side of the line.

Responsible parents used to keep tabs on their kids but were not involved with them. They knew the where, what, and with whom of their children's lives, but they maintained a respectful distance, letting their kids learn the hard way, by trial and error.

In this context, the child's primary challenge was to keep his parents from getting involved. He eventually figured out that the way to bring about minimal "government" intrusion into his life was to act responsibly. His parents got involved when he failed to act responsibly, the consequence of which was less freedom. It didn't take many such episodes of parental involvement for him to "get it."

Parenting is a form of leadership. In order for a leader to be effective, he or she must command, as opposed to demand, the respect of the people being led. This requires a boundary between the leader and the led. Getting involved with your kids puts relationship before leadership, the cart before the horse. It often results in the distinction between parents and children being blurred, turning the parents into quasi-peers, and making it difficult for the children to accept the parents' authority. Whining, petulance, and problems with discipline are the likely outcome.

High involvement transitions all too easily into micromanagement, in which case the child quickly learns that if he drops the proverbial ball, his parents will not just pick it up, but probably also clean it up. They may even begin carrying it for him. As he becomes more dependent on his parent' rescuing, he begins acting less and less capable. In turn, his parents become ever more convinced that he requires their constant vigilance—their involvement—in order to succeed. The parents end up working harder and harder to ensure the success of a child who is working hardly at all, which is why highly involved parents are likely to be highly stressed parents as well.

In addition, parents who are highly involved in things like their children's homework begin to take their children's successes and failures personally. They end up preventing most of the error in the trial and error process and cleaning up those errors that do slip by them. The result being that the child fails to learn important life lessons.

That's why I think parental involvement, *as I define it*, is bad for both parents and children.

The other day after my wife returned home from taking our youngest daughters to school, she said to me, "There was a father at school and he was carrying his little daughter's book pack." You might be thinking, *Well, that father was very thoughtful.* I would agree if for some reason that little girl could not physically carry her own book pack; but that wasn't the case.

I love all my children; but I have long held that one of the most important things you can teach your children is how to work so they won't become an entitlement child. This is one of the reasons we are a fat nation and have too many fat children. Teaching your children to work brings happiness to them. They may not think so when they are being taught how to work, but later they will thank you. That's the NAKED TRUTH.

Some dads and many mothers exist in a very stressful environment because they feel a need to get their little ones involved in everything everyone else has their kids involved in. Talk about peer pressure.

We all need to get back to nature to the call of the wild where you can hear the birds chirping, the squirrels chattering, the sound of the camp fire crackling, see the sun rise on a crisp spring morning, or see the sun setting in the west.

Right now, it is 5:28 A.M. CST April 20, 2011 as I'm writing and I have the door to my apartment open enough to hear the birds chirping. It is still dark and it's raining, I can hear the roar of the thunder and I see the lightning. I don't have a television to distract me. No one is here except me. It's nice. I get up early every day and yes, even on the weekend. Many people say "I'm going to sleep in on the weekend" and sometimes they will not crawl out of bed before noon and usually that's because during the week they have gone to bed late every night but yet had to get up and go to work the next morning.

Your body and mind have been wonderfully and marvelously created by God. You have a biological clock that He has placed within you that is precise. The greatest thing your body and mind need is regularity and balance.

If you lay around on the weekends and get up late, you will be more tired on Monday mornings than if you get up earlier or near the same time you arise on any other day. You will find you can accomplish more in the early hours of the morning than you can in the late hours of the night. But you must go to bed earlier if you expect to rise early and feel rested and refreshed.

Remember every hour of sleep you get before midnight is really equal to two hours of sleep after midnight. This is the time the stress-lowering hormones are secreted and why you feel more refreshed and rested in the morning if you get more sleep before midnight. Don't let a television show or a movie you think you need to watch rob you of the sleep your mind and body need. These actors don't care a hoot about your well-being. Television can stifle your imagination and creativity, especially, in the very young.

The other day, my wife and I went to the store together, which doesn't happen very often. We immediately found a parking space because we park away from the store so we can have a greater distance for walking, plus the added benefit of not having any cars next to yours banging their doors into yours. But the real reason is to have a chance to walk. Purchase a pedometer.

A pedometer, a pager-sized device worn on your belt, simply records the number of steps you take based on your body's movement. You'll pay anywhere from $10 to $25 either online or from a sporting store. I would encourage you if you can afford it to buy the more expensive version of $25. Now, that's not a bad investment.

The best way to start with a pedometer is to place it on your belt or on your pants just over the hip area. For the next three days, don't change your routine and at the end of the day record how many steps you have taken. Divide this number by three and this is your baseline from which to start your walking exercise program.

Remember all the steps count that you take during the day. This is one of the reasons I park away from the store. Many times, I see people driving all around the parking lot searching for that close up almost at the door parking space when I am already in the store. Another advantage of parking away from the store is you may reduce your stress if you are that type of person who screams expletives or who uses sign language at someone who has just stolen your parking space. It amazes me how many people know sign language in the heat of the moment.

Last night, as I was leaving Wal-Mart, I noticed one of the greeters explaining to a woman about thirty years old how to use one of those powered shopping carts that you drive around in. She looked to be over-weight but not excessively. Now I can't say if she had some underlying neurological disease that I couldn't see, but she was moving about pretty freely before she mounted the motorized shopping cart. She had four family members or friends that were with her who could assist her if she needed help.

The argument I am presenting here is to walk whenever and wherever you have the opportunity.

So with your new pedometer and working from your baseline, have a goal of finally walking 10,000 steps a day. That would be about four miles. If you're walking briskly, you probably have a stride of between two and a half to three feet, so 2,000 steps is about a mile.

Walking still remains the single best exercise you can begin; an exercise program that doesn't cost you a penny, but that gives you the biggest return for your investment. Many times when people want to lose weight, they decide they are going to start out running and within a few days to a few weeks or months they end up with plantar fasciitis; and then they face the prospect of not being able to run or even walk for weeks to months.

Plantar fasciitis is such an easy injury to avoid but it happens in a lot of people who are just starting or who are getting back into an exercise program.

And many people after experiencing a plantar fasciitis, get so discouraged, because it can take from weeks or even months to heal, that they just simply give up.

But I want to encourage you to never give up. Remember, there is no such thing as failure. You don't fail at anything, you just quit before the finish line. And this is true with anything in your life. If you don't quit, it's impossible to fail. So keep looking forward, not backward; keep focused up, not down, and you will gain the victory in whatever goal you are striving to achieve in making some simple lifestyle changes. Remember to set goals that are achievable for yourself otherwise you may become overloaded with stress and become depressed. Remember you can't fail in life as long as you don't quit; but you have failed already if you quit. When you were just a little baby you had to crawl before you could walk and then you had to walk before you could run and before you could ride a bike; but you didn't stop at crawling because you fell a few times or hundreds of times; no, you kept going until you could walk, run, ride a bike until those things were just a natural part of your life.

Well, that's how it is with making some simple lifestyle changes in your life. Don't ever give up. Don't look back; look ahead and pretty soon, you will be living a new lifestyle just as naturally as you walk; and you will be able to walk with a new spring in your step.

I recently spoke to a class of graduate students at Middle Tennessee School of Anesthesia because I am the president of the school's alumni. I knew they didn't want to hear me speak for long, because after I spoke they were finished and ready to leave. I told them that life can be like driving down an interstate. If you stay focused on the road ahead of you looking out the big windshield you have quite a view; but if you decide, like I did on a very straight stretch of highway, to see how long you can look into the rear view mirror and still remain on the road, you may end up in an accident. I don't recommend you do that. Well, that's how life is. If you remain with your eyes looking ahead of you, you will probably have a much safer trip; but if you begin looking back at only the sad and regrettable times in your life, then many times you'll find yourself feeling depressed.

The big word for a successful lifestyle change program is consistency. You can think of this as a motif. Consistency should be the thread or fiber that runs through every part of your lifestyle change program. Whatever program you start with and develop, be consistent and steadfast to it. Stay the course.

Your body develops muscle memory in everything you do and this is why regularity is so important to having good health.

It is good sometimes just to go back to the journal diary you kept for yourself that I wrote about in chapter two, and see how far you have progressed.

The human body is a marvelous machine and if properly taken care of, even without a warranty, it can serve you for many years, and someday for eternity.

And the good news is the warranty for your new marvelous machine doesn't cost you a dime except for time. And if you can't afford the time to exercise, then you need to begin right now today to rearrange your schedule because if you don't, you're not going to be around to even have a schedule, because you're going to be pushing daisies.

I have included here a fantastic article from the Mayo Clinic I found online.

Plantar Fasciitis - Topic Overview
Healthwise

CONTENT PROVIDED BY
MayoClinic.com

Plantar fasciitis—Comprehensive overview covers causes, prevention, self-care of this common type of heel pain.

Definition

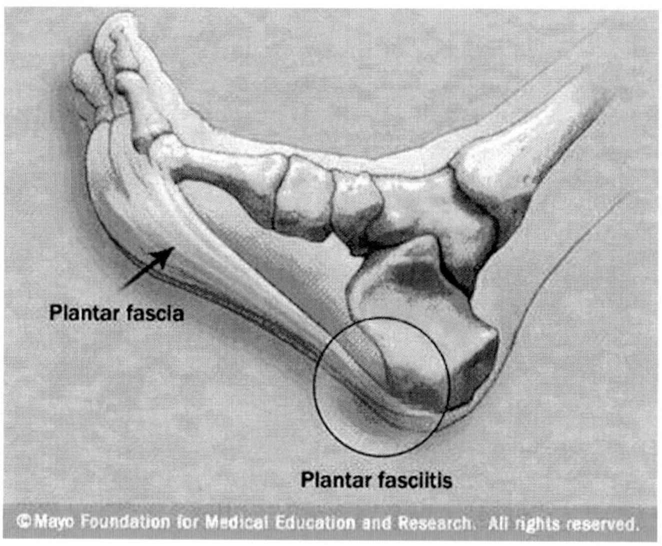

Plantar fasciitis is an inflammation of the fibrous tissue (plantar fascia) along the bottom of your foot that connects your heel bone to your toes. Plantar fasciitis can cause intense heel pain.

Plantar fasciitis (PLAN-tur fas-e-I-tis) is one of the most common causes of heel pain. It involves pain and inflammation of a thick band of tissue, called the plantar fascia, which runs across the bottom of your foot—connecting your heel bone to your toes.

Plantar fasciitis causes stabbing pain that usually occurs with your very first steps in the morning. Once your foot limbers up, the pain of plantar fasciitis normally decreases, but it may return after long periods of standing or after getting up from a seated position. Plantar fasciitis is particularly common in runners, people who are overweight, women who are pregnant. Those who wear shoes with inadequate support are at a higher risk of plantar fasciitis.

Symptoms

In most cases, the pain associated with plantar fasciitis:

Develops gradually, affects just one foot, although it can occur in both feet simultaneously, is worst with the first few steps after awakening, although it also can be triggered by long periods of standing or getting up from a seated position, and feels like a sharp pain in the heel of your foot.

Under normal circumstances, your plantar fascia acts like a shock-absorbing bowstring supporting the arch in your foot. But if tension on that bowstring becomes too great, it can create small tears in the fascia. Repetitive stretching and tearing can cause the fascia to become irritated or inflamed.

Risk factors

Factors that may increase your risk of developing plantar fasciitis include:

Age. Plantar fasciitis is most common between the ages of forty and sixty.

Sex. Women are more likely than men to develop plantar fasciitis.

Certain types of exercise. Activities that place a lot of stress on your heel and attached tissue—such as long-distance running, ballet dancing, and dance aerobics—can contribute to an earlier onset of plantar fasciitis.

Faulty foot mechanics. Being flat-footed, having a high arch or even having an abnormal pattern of walking can adversely affect the way weight is distributed when you're standing, putting added stress on the plantar fascia.

Obesity. Excess pounds put extra stress on your plantar fascia.

Occupations that keep you on your feet. People with occupations that require a lot of walking or standing on hard surfaces—such as factory workers, teachers, and waitresses—can damage their plantar fascia.

Improper shoes. Shoes that are thin soled, loose, or lack arch support or the ability to absorb shock don't protect your feet. If you regularly wear shoes with high heels, your Achilles tendon—which is attached to your heel—can contract and shorten, causing strain on the tissue around your heel.

Complications

Ignoring plantar fasciitis may result in a chronic condition that hinders your regular activities. You may also develop foot, knee, hip, or back problems because of the way plantar fasciitis changes your walking motion.

Plantar fasciitis is an inflammation of the fibrous tissue (plantar fascia) along the bottom of your foot that connects your heel bone to your toes. Plantar fasciitis can cause intense heel pain.

Under normal circumstances, your plantar fascia acts like a shock-absorbing bowstring, supporting the arch in your foot. But, if tension on that bowstring becomes too great, it can create small tears in the fascia. Repetitive stretching and tearing can cause the fascia to become irritated or inflamed."

The Mandarin Duck: When we serve food especially fruits and vegetables, we need a variety of colors that will be inviting to the eye. When you prepare meals, have a variety of foods and a variety of colors; this will make the mealtime more inviting and satisfying.

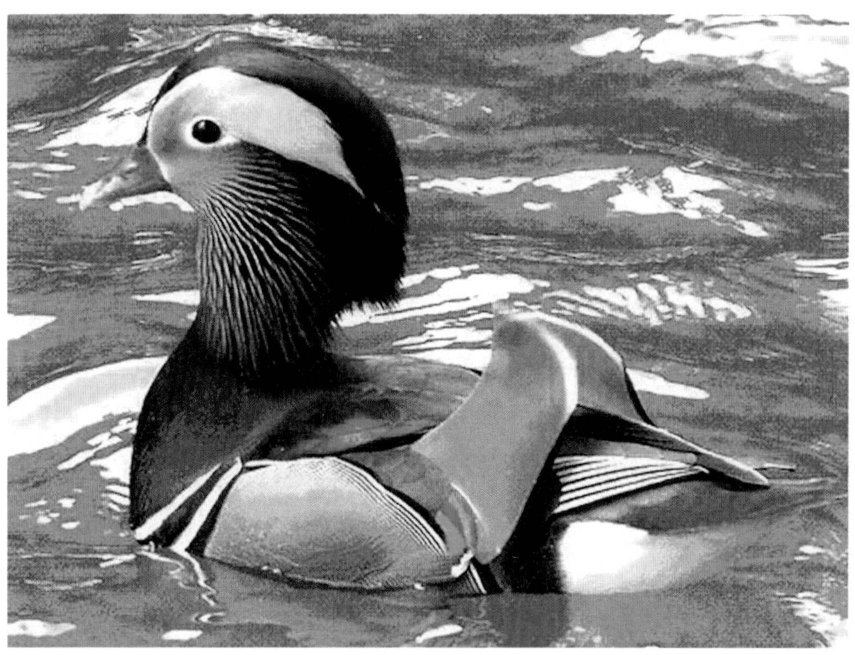

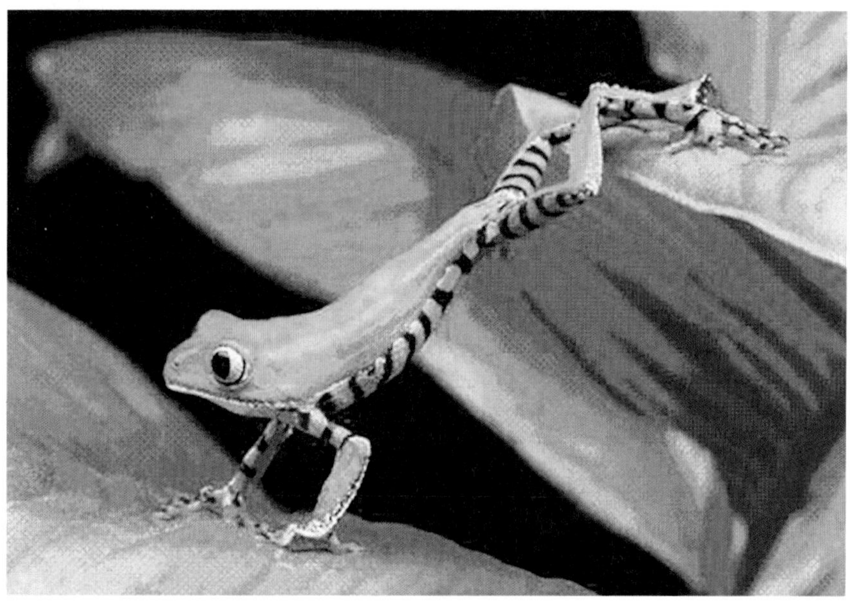

We should feel as good as the mandarin duck looks and be as agile as the tiger frog.

What do cats and dogs and most animals do when they first wake up? They go through a ritual of stretching. Both cats and dogs stretch their front paws way out in front of them. It's just instinct for them.

But if we start each day with a ritual of stretching and be consistent with it, in about three weeks it will almost become instinct to us. For humans, we call this making a habit out of it. It takes about twenty-one days or three weeks to form a new habit and then you don't even have to think about what you will do when you first wake up.

Always try to go to bed early like our grandmas did and get up early. There is a whole new world to see in the early hours of the morning. Each morning is new and fresh with no mistakes in it. Your attitude decides what kind of day you are going to have. If you choose to be happy and keep that perspective all the day long, you will be happy. After supper, many people sit around and watch television to make mush out of their minds. They have now been robbed of their imagination and creativity, and they will toss and turn more while they sleep since they stayed up and watched television. Before you retire to bed at night, your mind needs some quiet repose, relaxation, and thoughtful meditation.

> Someone gave me an article that really sums up what I'm talking about. It was written by Lisa Collier Cool:
> Couch potatoes beware watching the tube for two to three hours a day or more is linked to higher rates of early death from all causes, according to new research published today in the *Journal of the American Medical Association* (JAMA). The culprit is the couch potato lifestyle that frequently accompanies excessive viewing, the researchers report. With the average American logging five hours a day in front of the tube, sitting is replacing exercise.

> TV viewing is associated with unhealthy eating, setting the stage for weight gain, the study indicates. Packing on pounds, in turn, boosts risk for diabetes, heart attacks, and a shorter life. Studies also link excessive tube time to sleep deprivation (another heart health hazard) and even nearsightedness in kids. Don't blame the TV—it can't shove you onto the couch or serve up a fast food meal. If your main form of physical activity is pushing buttons on the remote, take a look at how these habits can impact your health.

And many people eat something late to go along with their television watching. Eating late in the evening will add about two pounds per month to your body. Just think about it; if you quit eating in the evening you would lose at least two pounds per month—all other things being equal; so in one year you would have dropped twenty-four pounds without doing anything else.

When you lose weight slowly, you are mainly losing fat and not muscle which is what you want in any weight loss program. Muscle is the largest fat burning organ in the body so if you are losing muscle, your body will actually hang onto to fat thinking you are in a starvation mode. This again is why strength training is so important in making lifestyle changes.

Also remember when you lose weight quickly, you will most likely gain it back quickly and more besides, and you will end up worse than before you started a weight loss plan.

Stay away from all weight loss programs that tell you anything about losing weight quickly. It may happen but the weight you're losing initially is water and after that muscle and unfortunately fat often is the last poundage to be lost.

Remember, when you are starting on a program to slim down, don't go out and buy a scale, go and purchase a tape measure, because if you add strength training to your weight loss program, you may see a little weight gain, initially, but if you measure your waist you will see you have lost inches. Isn't that good news?

Chapter Nine: Depression

Most experts will agree that causes of depression fall into three categories:

- Genetics
- Environment
- Chemical imbalances in the brain

There are five major types of depression:

1. Unipolar
2. Dysthymia
3. Bipolar disorder or manic depressive
4. SAD Seasonal Affective Disorder
5. Post-partum depression

And finally, there is a depression that all of us will face at some time in our lives: when we lose a loved one or for anything we need to grieve for. Some call it grieving depression. It is very normal and is actually part of our grieving process. It's only when we continue to grieve and cannot turn away from that loss and we begin to lose hope that it can become a problem.

So many people are on antidepressant medications today but I truly feel they don't need to be. Quite honestly, an easy way to practice medicine is to just dole out the medications because today it is a numbers game. I work in surgery and I know that CEO's of hospitals and surgery centers have a quota that they expect to be met at the end of each month. And one of the most misused and wrongly prescribed medications are antidepressants.

Here is just a sample of what one pharmaceutical company says about one of their drugs, Cymbalta.

Indication

Cymbalta is indicated for the treatment of major depressive disorder (MDD). The efficacy of Cymbalta was established in four short-term and one maintenance trial in adults.
Cymbalta is indicated for the treatment of generalized anxiety disorder (GAD). The efficacy of Cymbalta was established in three short-term and one maintenance trial in adults.
Cymbalta is indicated for the management of diabetic peripheral neuropathic pain (DPNP) and fibromyalgia.

Important Safety Information About Cymbalta

Antidepressants can increase suicidal thoughts and behaviors in children, teens, and young adults. Suicide is a known risk of depression and some other psychiatric disorders. Call your doctor right away if you have new or worsening depression symptoms, unusual changes in behavior, or thoughts of suicide. Be especially observant within the first few months of treatment or after a change in dose. Approved only for adults 18 and over.

What should I talk about with my healthcare provider?

Patients on antidepressants and their families or caregivers should watch for new or worsening depression symptoms, unusual changes in behavior, thoughts of suicide, anxiety, agitation, panic attacks, difficulty sleeping, irritability, hostility, aggressiveness, impulsivity, restlessness, or extreme hyperactivity. Call your healthcare provider right away if you have thoughts of suicide or if any of these symptoms are severe or occur suddenly. Be especially observant within the first few months of antidepressant treatment or whenever there is a change in dose.

Who should NOT take Cymbalta?

You should not take Cymbalta if:
You have recently taken a type of antidepressant called a monoamine oxidase inhibitor (MAOI)
You have uncontrolled narrow-angle glaucoma (increased eye pressure)
You are taking Mellaril® (thioridazine)

What other important information should I discuss with my healthcare provider?

Before starting Cymbalta, talk with your healthcare provider:

- about all of your medical conditions, including kidney or liver problems, glaucoma, diabetes, seizures, or if you have bipolar disorder. Cymbalta may worsen a type of glaucoma or the control of blood sugar in some patients with diabetes
- about your alcohol use
- if you are taking nonprescription or prescription medicines, including those for migraine, to address a possible life-threatening condition

- ➢ if you are taking NSAID pain relievers, aspirin, or blood thinners. Use with Cymbalta may increase bleeding risk
- ➢ if you are pregnant, plan to become pregnant during therapy, or are breastfeeding an infant

While taking Cymbalta, talk with your healthcare provider:

- ➢ if you have itching, right upper belly pain, dark urine, yellow skin/eyes, or unexplained flu-like symptoms, which may be signs of liver problems. Severe liver problems, sometimes fatal, have been reported
- ➢ if you have high fever, confusion, and stiff muscles to address a possible life-threatening condition
- ➢ before stopping Cymbalta or changing your dose
- ➢ if you experience dizziness or fainting upon standing, especially when first starting Cymbalta or when increasing the dose
- ➢ about your blood pressure. Cymbalta can increase your blood pressure. Your healthcare provider should check your blood pressure prior to and while taking Cymbalta
- ➢ if you experience headache, weakness, confusion, problems concentrating, memory problems, or feel unsteady while taking Cymbalta which may be signs of low sodium levels
- ➢ if you develop problems with urine flow

If you have any questions, talk to your healthcare provider before taking Cymbalta.

What are the possible side effects of Cymbalta?

The most common side effect of Cymbalta was nausea. Other common side effects included dry mouth, constipation, sleepiness, increased sweating, decreased appetite, dizziness, and weakness. This is not a complete list of side effects.

Other safety information about Cymbalta:

Cymbalta may cause sleepiness and dizziness. Until you know how Cymbalta affects you, you should not drive a car or operate hazardous machinery.

Wow! After reading about all the warnings and who shouldn't be taking this drug, do you really want to take this drug for anything? Now, this isn't the only drug on the market with these kinds of warnings. I chose Cymbalta because they have a clear and succinct ad especially when it comes to the warnings and contraindications of the drug. They are just trying to protect their companies from lawsuits.

I knew a lady who was suffering from depression whose son was a doctor. She wouldn't get out of her house and her depression was getting worse. One day, the son told his mother, "You need to get out of the house and start walking."

That's great advice and that is where I like to start with any patient experiencing depression, to get them to start walking. I'm not talking about doing it for cardio training; no, I want them to walk and breathe in deeply and take in the nature all around them and just have a relaxing and refreshing walk. Follow the squirrels as they chase each other about and as they jump from limb to limb and from tree to tree. Listen to the birds and get to know the song of the different birds. Smell the flowers along the way. Just the other day, I was walking in my neighborhood and noticed a beautiful flower and wondered if the flower had any scent. I moved closer and sniffed a little and found out that flower didn't have any odor at all; but as I took the time to pause and investigate about that flower, well, just for a moment I didn't have a care in the world; it was refreshing.

Distance isn't the key, at first, when you begin a walking program. I know some people when they walk it's all about going as fast as they can and covering a certain distance even if it kills them—and it may if they don't have the right attitude. Not always, but often, we bring our type "A" personalities even into our recovery phase of the lifestyle changes we are attempting to institute; and many times, that is what got us there in the first place.

I'm reminded of a song actually entitled "59th St. Bridge Song," by artists Simon and Garfunkel that really paints a picture of what I am trying to share.

Slow down, you move too fast.
You got to make the morning last.
Just kicking down the cobble stones.
Looking for fun and feelin' groovy.
Hello lamppost,
What cha knowing?
I've come to watch your flowers growing.
Ain't cha got no rhymes for me?
Doot-in' doo-doo,
Feelin' groovy.

Got no deeds to do,
No promises to keep.
I'm dappled and drowsy and ready to sleep.
Let the morning time drop all its petals on me.
Life, I love you,
All is groovy.

I had dinner with a retired radiologist and his wife and, while other people were there, I was explaining to this woman the dangers of taking drugs like Cymbalta long term. The radiologist who is in his 70's said "I've been on Cymbalta for about fifteen years. I've tried coming off Cymbalta and had bad feelings about committing suicide; I'll be on this drug for the rest of life."

This is really just what the drug cartels want—your total dependence upon one of their life destroying drugs for the rest of your life. In this case, instead of having a physical dependence with things like alcohol, or tobacco, you have a mental or psychological dependence with your feelings. It's like having a third conscience that's encouraging you to do bad things like committing suicide.

Another friend of mine who has a doctorate in education, at the time, had been on antidepressants for over seventeen years. One day, he and I were traveling on the Los Angeles freeway headed to his house in Palm Springs at 120 miles an hour. Just then, he said to me, "Sometimes I feel I just want to turn the steering wheel real sharp to the right and end everything."

These are really sad stories about real people educated and not educated, young and old, rich and poor, but most of them are caught in the web of seeking treatment for their depression through prescription drugs—the legal kind.

Walking is still one of the best exercises that doesn't cost a dime, helps clear your mind, starts the blood circulating, lowers cholesterol, lowers blood pressure, stabilizes your blood sugar, gives you a healthier attitude, lowers stress, and makes you look better, especially if you walk outside. If it's possible, always do your walking outside where you can breathe in fresh air. When you go to a gym or are at home walking on a treadmill you are really breathing stale air. So if you must walk on a treadmill for safety or convenience or for whatever reason you can't walk outside, then make sure you have your windows open to receive fresh air. Having plants inside really helps because they take up the carbon dioxide or wastes that we exhale.

Proper breathing is very important when you are walking. Take deep breathes in through your nose with your mouth closed and exhale through your mouth. Try to inhale and exhale slowly. If you have a sedentary job, make sure you practice proper breathing while sitting. No one around you will even know you are breathing deeply unless you tell them and that's always a good idea to share lifestyle ideas that are helping you. You will be more alert at work and you will not need all that coffee and those soft drinks to keep you awake. When I get sleepy at work, I will drink some water, inhale and exhale deeply, and if possible get up and stretch or take a few steps. You will be more productive in whatever work you are doing. When I'm driving and I become sleepy, I will go through some deep breathing exercises and if I need to I will pull over, get out, and walk around and do some stretches.

And what's amazing is you just feel better mentally and it doesn't cost you a dime and you didn't take any drugs to make you stay awake.

Remember the Mandarin duck picture with all the beautiful array of colors; well, the following article on combating health problems with exercise incorporates a lot of color which just may encourage us to exercise.

Seven Ways to Combat Health Problems with Exercise

Reduce pain, fight depression, slow osteoporosis, and other ways to use exercise for a healthier life.

By Linda Melone for *MSN Health & Fitness*

Content provided by:

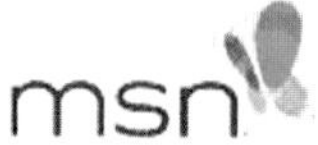

1 of 8

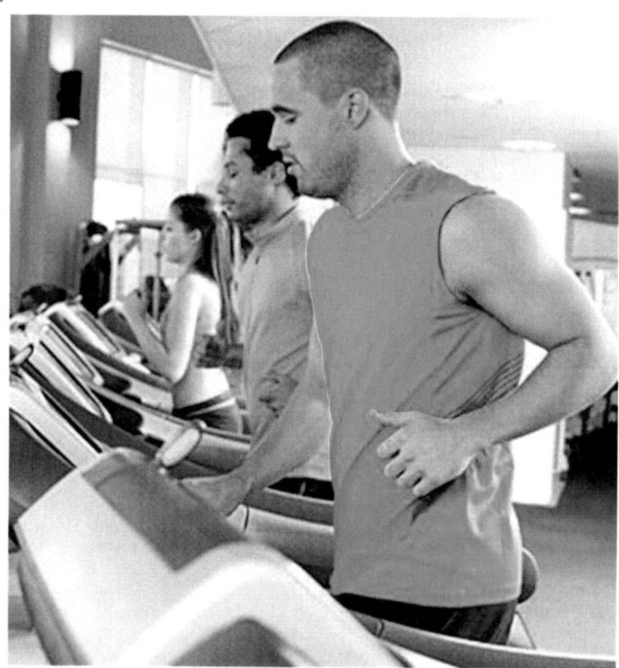

Endorphins and Your Mood

Ever notice how much better you feel when you exercise after a stressful day? It's more than just psychological, says David Geier, Jr., MD, sports medicine director of the Medical University of South Carolina. "Exercise kicks in natural brain chemicals called endorphins that elevate your mood." And that's just the beginning. "Exercise is good for all kinds of health problems," says Dr. Geier. Read on for ways to add to or alter your current exercise program to maximize benefits for what ails you.

Seven Ways to Combat Health Problems with Exercise

Reduce pain, fight depression, slow osteoporosis, and other ways to use exercise for a healthier life.

By Linda Melone for *MSN Health & Fitness*

Content provided by:

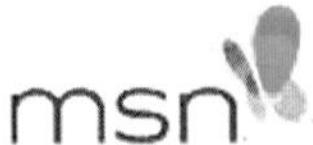

2 of 8

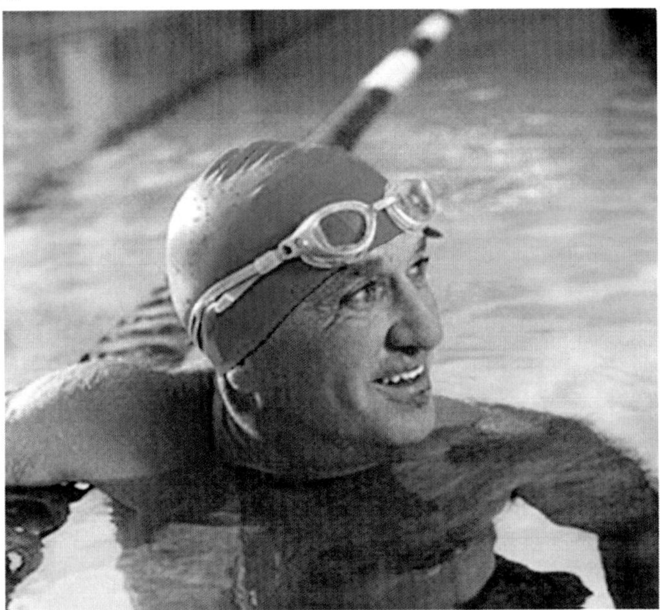

Arthritis? Just Add Water

Movement helps achy joints feel less achy, but getting started can be tough when you hurt. If exercising on land is too uncomfortable, seek out a pool. Water provides twelve times the resistance of air, so you strengthen muscles without stressing your joints.

Also consider other ways to modify your current routine. If you're on a treadmill, for example, raise the incline to increase the challenge instead of jogging or running, which can impact joints. Plan to exercise later in the day if you wake up with painful joints. Be sure to warm up thoroughly by taking a hot bath or shower and/or starting out slowly. Keep in mind the two-hour rule: "If you still hurt two hours after exercise, cut back on the intensity," says Nutting.

Seven Ways to Combat Health Problems with Exercise

Reduce pain, fight depression, slow osteoporosis, and other ways to use exercise for a healthier life.

By Linda Melone for *MSN Health & Fitness*

Content provided by:

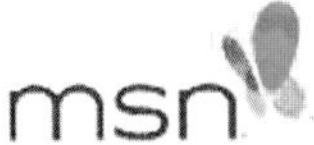

3 of 8

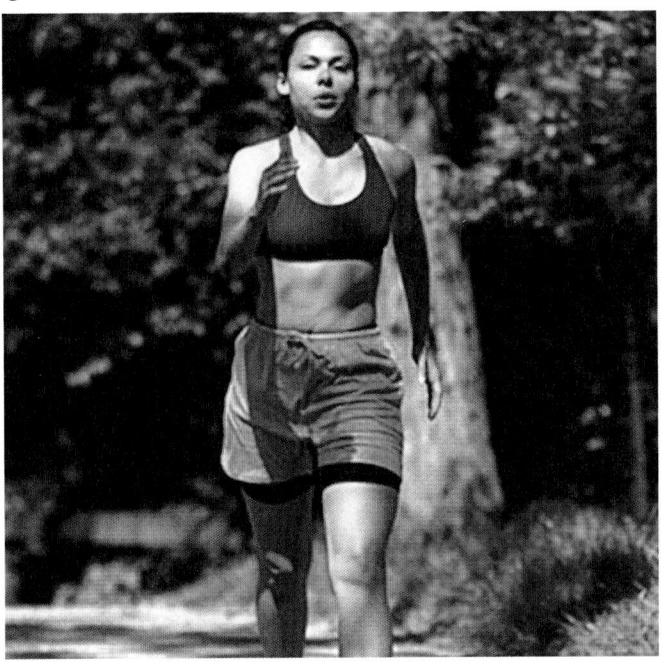

Headaches? Breathe Easy

If you're leaving work with a headache from a hectic day and heading to the gym, take a few minutes to relax, says Karilee H. Shames PhD, RN, author of *Feeling Fat, Fuzzy, or Frazzled?* (Hudson Street Press, 2005) and a certified clinical specialist in psychiatric nursing and in holistic nursing. "Sit in your car or other quiet place and do some slow deep breathing before you go into a noisy gym." Or consider skipping the gym and walking outdoors in nature or walking on a home treadmill instead (if home is quieter).

If you enjoy walking, try picking up the pace, says Naheed Ali, MD, author of *Are You Fit To Live? 4 Steps to Improving Your Health* (SabellaPress, 2009) and a faculty member of The Pennsylvania Institute of Technology. "Speed walking loosens you up and allows for much better circulation throughout all regions of the body, including the brain," says Dr. Ali.

Seven Ways to Combat Health Problems with Exercise

Reduce pain, fight depression, slow osteoporosis, and other ways to use exercise for a healthier life.
By Linda Melone for *MSN Health & Fitness*

Content provided by:

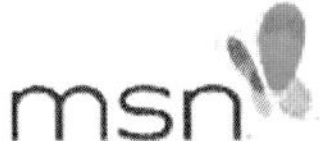

4 of 8

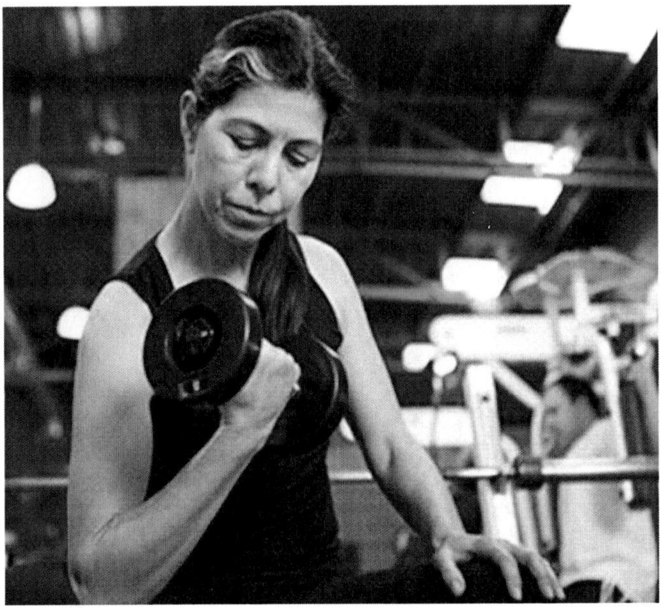

Osteoporosis? Up the Weights

If your last *bone mineral scan* was less than optimal, resistance training can help stimulate bone growth. "Any exercise is good," says Geier. "But focus on weight bearing or resistance training. Even light resistance in addition to walking has some impact." The most effective exercises work multiple joints, such as the squat [1]. Keep in mind, however, that an exercise affects only the bone(s) involved in the move, says Mark Nutting, CSCS, NSCA personal trainer of the year 2009, of Saco Sport and Fitness, Maine. "So exercises that strengthen your legs, hips, and spine won't benefit your wrists," says Nutting. Strive for a full body resistance program focusing on large muscle groups. Include squats and overhead shoulder presses, which strengthen the bones most often weakened by osteoporosis.

Seven Ways to Combat Health Problems with Exercise

Reduce pain, fight depression, slow osteoporosis, and other ways to use exercise for a healthier life.
By Linda Melone for *MSN Health & Fitness*

Content provided by:

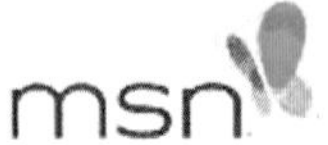

5 of 8

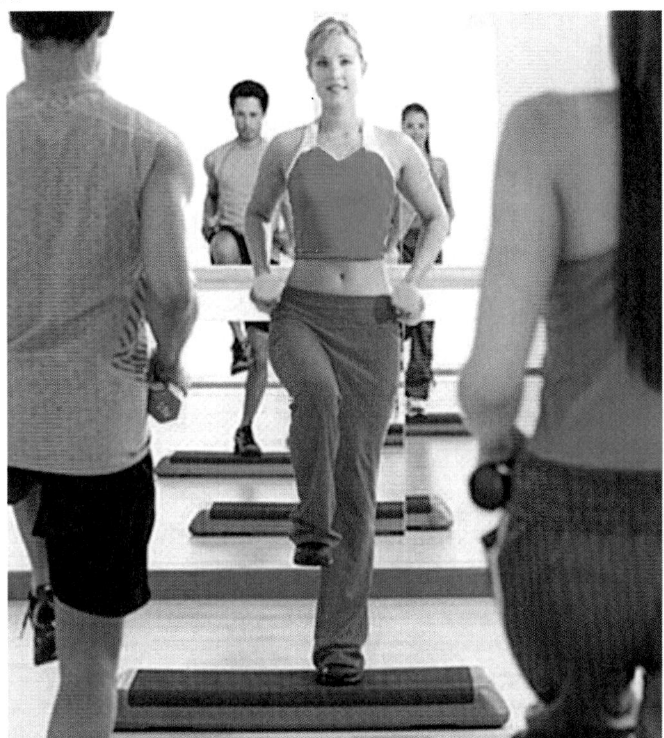

Depressed? Get Moving

Feeling down? Join a class or go for a run. "Mild exercise is effective to a certain extent against virtually any form of depression," says Dr. Ali. "But more intense movement and exercise can be carried out if you've been working out consistently for a long period of time. Being around other people can help lift your mood as well, especially if loneliness brings on depression."

Join an exercise class or a running or walking club. You'll combine the physical benefits of exercise with the psychological lift of social interaction. Or go for a long run. Runners often report a euphoric state called a "runner's high" after running long distances [2]. "Cardiovascular exercise is most likely to release the feel-good neurotransmitters (brain chemicals) and trigger a 'high,'" says Geier.

Seven Ways to Combat Health Problems with Exercise

Reduce pain, fight depression, slow osteoporosis, and other ways to use exercise for a healthier life.
By Linda Melone for *MSN Health & Fitness*

Content provided by:

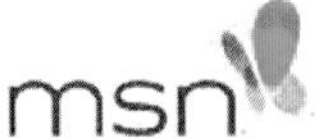

6 of 8

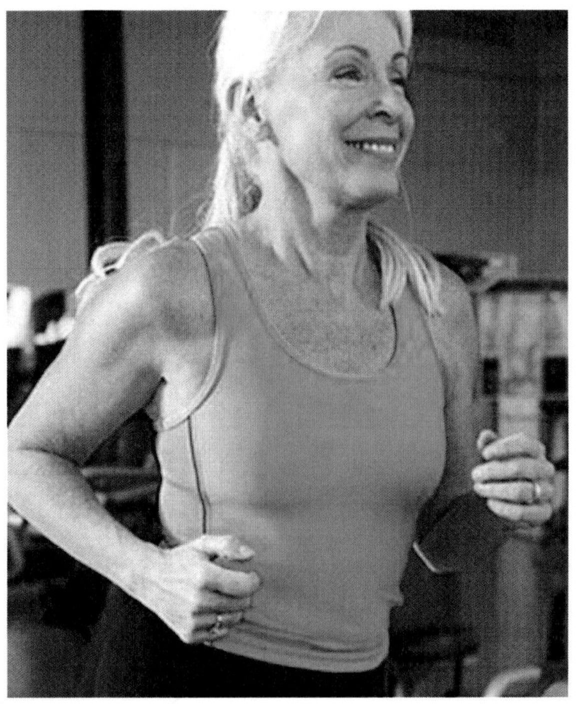

Menopausal? Combine Weights and Cardio

Keep active by lifting weights and performing cardiovascular exercise and you'll be less likely to gain weight after menopause. Hormonal changes and a drop in muscle mass during menopause can make it harder to lose weight, which often accumulates around the abdominal area. "Weight lifting increases muscle mass and keeps your metabolism stoked," says Geier. "Resistance exercise two to three times a week also helps keep bones strong and reduces your risk of osteoporosis after menopause." Add regular walking, swimming, biking, or other cardiovascular activity thirty minutes, five days a week or perform three ten-minute mini exercise bouts to reap the same health benefits, as recommended by the American College of Sports Medicine.

Seven Ways to Combat Health Problems with Exercise

Reduce pain, fight depression, slow osteoporosis, and other ways to use exercise for a healthier life.
By Linda Melone for MSN Health & Fitness

Content provided by:

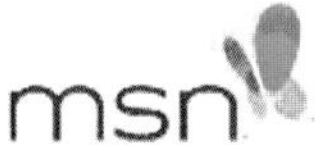

7 of 8

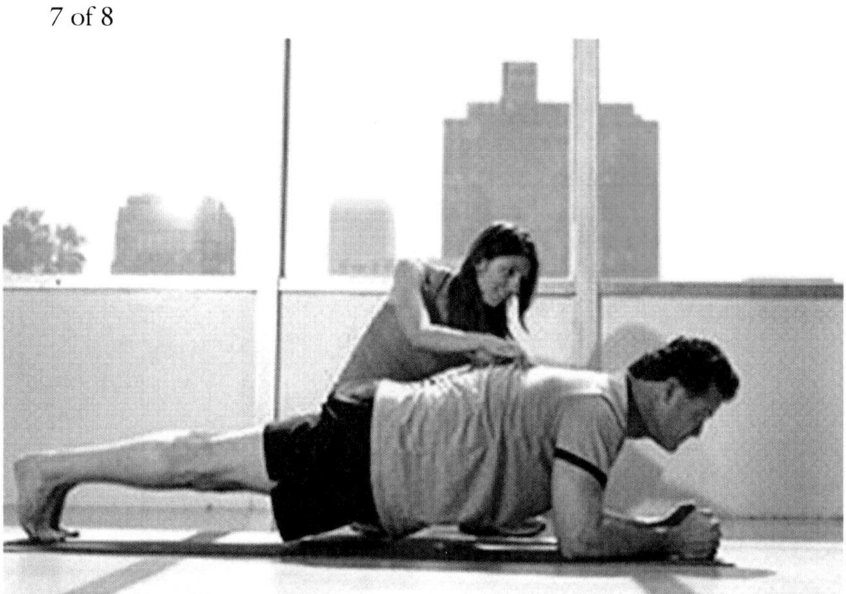

Back Pain? Work the Core

Poor posture and weak core, back or abdominal muscles can add up to back pain. "You need to develop the strength and ability to stabilize your spine and keep it in proper alignment while doing activities," says Nutting. "Practice good posture and learn how to properly engage your core muscles." The best core strengthener: the plank. Lie on your stomach on an exercise mat with your elbows close to your sides and directly under your shoulders, palms down. Contract your core and abdominal muscles. Slowly lift your entire torso off the floor or mat, maintaining a stiff torso and legs. Avoid any arching or sagging of your low back or hiking (upwards) in your hips, holding this position for twenty seconds or longer. Add this to your exercise routine two to three times a week, working up to sixty seconds. Raise one leg off the ground for a greater challenge.

Seven Ways to Combat Health Problems with Exercise

Reduce pain, fight depression, slow osteoporosis, and other ways to use exercise for a healthier life.
By Linda Melone for MSN Health & Fitness

Content provided by:

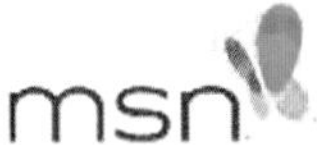

8 of 8

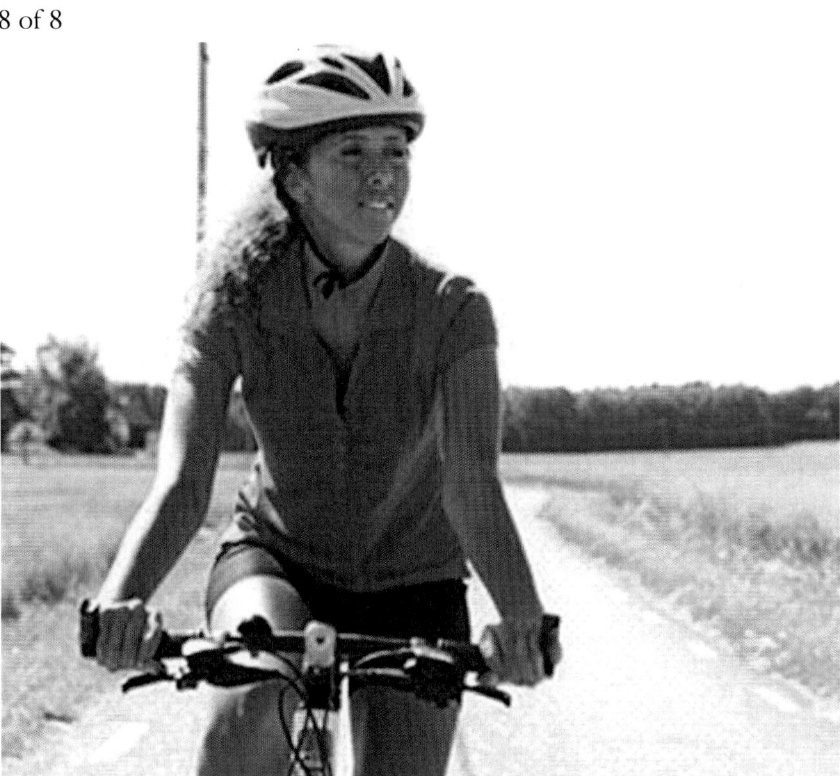

Fibromyalgia or Chronic Pain? Slow and Steady

Motivating yourself to exercise can be difficult when you're in chronic pain. And, unlike arthritis, symptoms of fibromyalgia can vary from day to day and pain may affect different muscles as well. "What works for one person with fibromyalgia may not work for another," says Geier. Be sure to warm up thoroughly, start easy, and use long rest periods. "If you overdo, it can take a long time to recover," says Geier. Start with as few as three to five minutes and work your way up to twenty minutes or longer by adding one to two minutes at a time.

Try various activities such as walking, swimming (look for facilities with heated pools), and biking. *Recumbent bikes* offer more back support and may be preferable to uprights. Start slowly, progress gradually, and be consistent.

Improper management of our time is one of the most common causes of depression. You get up in the morning and by evening time, you are discouraged because you didn't accomplish what you expected you should have. The good news is it doesn't cost you a dime to start managing your time better. Well, it may if you feel you need professional help and that's okay, too, to get you started in the right direction.

One of the things I try to do each day is set goals (short term and long-term goals) of what I want to accomplish. You have to make sure your goals are reasonable or at the least achievable. Always make sure you set smaller very easily achievable goals each day. This will bring you some immediate sense of accomplishment and a feeling of success. It's like when you are in debt and you begin paying off your smaller bills and then start debt rolling to your larger bills that you see you have actually paid off a bill. It is amazing what that does for your attitude.

You may not get through but one of the goals you set for yourself for that day, but that's okay. Give yourself a pat on the back at the end of the day. You really made some progress. You set goals and followed through by successfully completing at least one. Now, follow that same plan the next day and pretty soon you have formed a habit and you will notice very quickly how good you feel about yourself. Being organized, setting goals, and finally reaching those goals really does change your attitude.

One way to assure you reach your goals and continue to be successful is to learn to say no when your plate is full. And it might be a very good thing you have to say no, too. But the only way in which to know your plate is full is to have goals set and a plan to accomplish them. Plan your work and then work your plan.

One of the hardest lessons I had to learn about saying no was it was all right to say no to nominating committees when I was asked to serve in some position at our church. Unfortunately, the statistics haven't changed much when it comes to church work. Twenty percent of the people still do eighty percent of the work and are responsible for eighty percent of the giving.

Because I have, for the most part, a choleric/sanguine personality, many times I just say yes to some request without even thinking about the long term ramifications; or I will accept some invite to someone's house for dinner after church without even talking it over with my wife.

> Both the hummingbird and the vulture fly over our nation's deserts. All vultures see is rotting meat, because that is what they look for. They thrive on that diet. But hummingbirds ignore the smelly flesh of dead animals. Instead, they look for the colorful blossoms of desert plants. The vultures live on what was. They live on the past. They fill themselves with what is dead and gone. But hummingbirds live on what is. They seek new life. They fill themselves with freshness and life. Each bird finds what it is looking for. We all do.

Steve Goodier, *Quote* Magazine, in *Reader's Digest*, May, 1990.

Everything in life has to do with mind over matter, especially when it comes to making even simple lifestyle changes.

I was listening to an interview on 3ABN (Three Angels Broadcasting Network), a Christian television station and the president of 3ABN ask the man he was interviewing about his age. I believe he was in his seventies. He said, "If you don't mind, it doesn't matter how old you are."

Don't let anyone or anything steal your joy. If you are in a battle with depression, and that's what it is, you are probably looking through eyes that give you a jaded slant to everything you take in, particularly when it comes to relationships.

When you get up in the morning each day, check your pulse and if you find you have one, then understand you have a purpose in life for that day. Don't worry about what happened yesterday, except for the good times, because you can't change yesterday, it's gone forever; and don't fret about tomorrow for it hasn't arrived. There will be enough for you to deal within your life for one day. We can learn from our mistakes from yesterday and remain determined that we will not make those same mistakes again; but if we do, and we all will, that's okay, just don't dwell on the past.

Each day I pray for peace when reflecting on the past, grace and faith for the present, and finally glory and hope for the future. I can guarantee you, from personal experience, that prayer will always be answered.

I like that gospel song "One day at a time sweet Jesus that's all I've asking from you, help me today, show me the way one day at a time." I don't know anyone that has found or has true happiness because of the things they have; it is quite the opposite. We should love people and use things, but many times, we end up loving things and using people. When we use people, relationships are placed in jeopardy and we may find ourselves depressed.

For most Americans, our focus and goals are at the end of the journey of life and so we work hard all our lives, invest heavily, burn the candle at both ends, and prepare for a great retirement of playing golf or whatever it is you like to do. The problem isn't the preparation for the retirement, preparation is always a good thing; the issue is our health usually suffers because we have neglected to take time to stay healthy. Now all the money we have worked for and saved is going for prescriptions, CAT scans, surgeries (many times not needed), and a whole slew of other treatments paid out for medical needs. The Eastern mind has a little different mindset; they enjoy the journey, so they stop and smell the roses. They don't care so much about money as they do their health. They do look forward at times I suppose to their retirement, but it is not the all-encompassing thing in their lives.

When my father-in-law passed away in 1984 as a patient in Florida Hospital in Orlando, Florida, there were a lot of medical bills. It took most of my mother-in-law's savings to pay all those medical bills. That is downright sad.

Following are twelve famous people who suffered with depression.

Content provided by: msn

< Previous | Next >

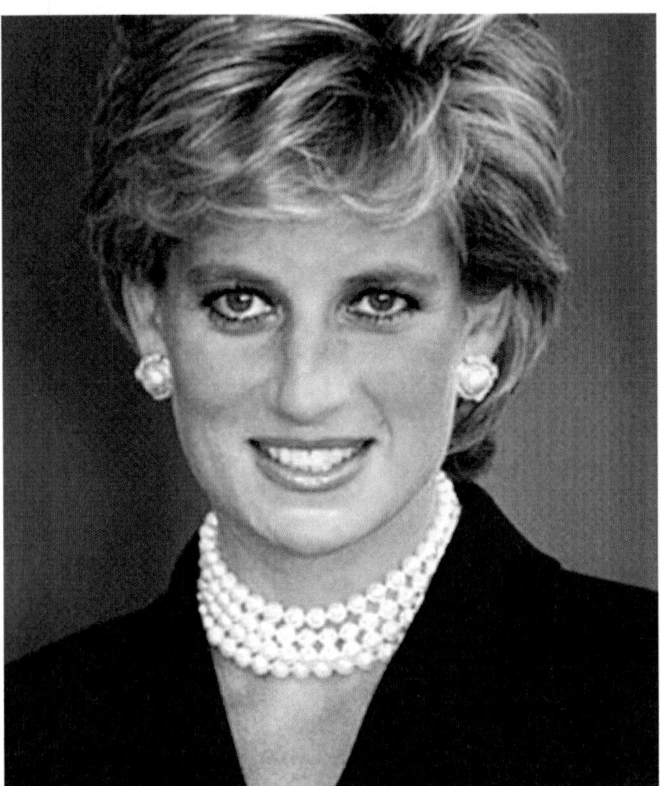

Diana, Princess of Wales

Diana herself referred to the early years of her royal life as "the dark ages," and it's not difficult to believe the young Princess of Wales was smiling shyly through significant pain. Biographers detail how Diana's inner life was perpetually at odds with what her public life required. Her depression and anxiety took several forms, including bulimia nervosa, postpartum depression after the birth of son, William, and numerous "cries for help" that included pen-knife cuts to her chest and thighs and slashes to her wrists with a razor.

Through it all, Diana lived as an inspiration to millions and was widely praised for her far-reaching charity work. The Princess of Wales remains one of the best-loved figures of the twentieth century.

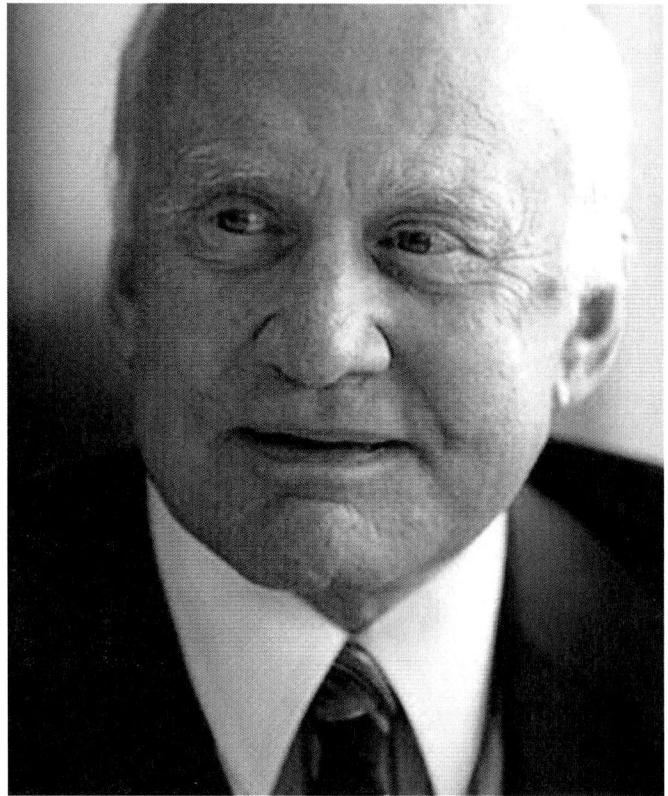

Buzz Aldrin

It was a long way down for astronaut Buzz Aldrin. The second man ever to set foot on the moon was retired from NASA in 1972—a change that stripped his life of purpose and direction, according to his 2009 autobiography, *Magnificent Desolation*. Relentless media attention further contributed to Aldrin's descent, and he found himself consumed by depression and alcoholism. He also knew that depression had a genetic component, and feared that he could follow in the suicidal steps of his grandfather and his mother, Marion Moon Aldrin.

With help, Aldrin recovered and recommitted himself to promoting the exploration of space. A recent television cameo provides some evidence of Aldrin's health—and his ability to laugh at himself. On a Mother's Day episode of 30 Rock, Buzz lists the many personal demons he has conquered and then yells victoriously at the moon, "I walked on your face!"

Inspirational, In Spite of Depression

Great thinkers, artists, leaders, and explorers alike who have inspired us, even in the face of severe depression.

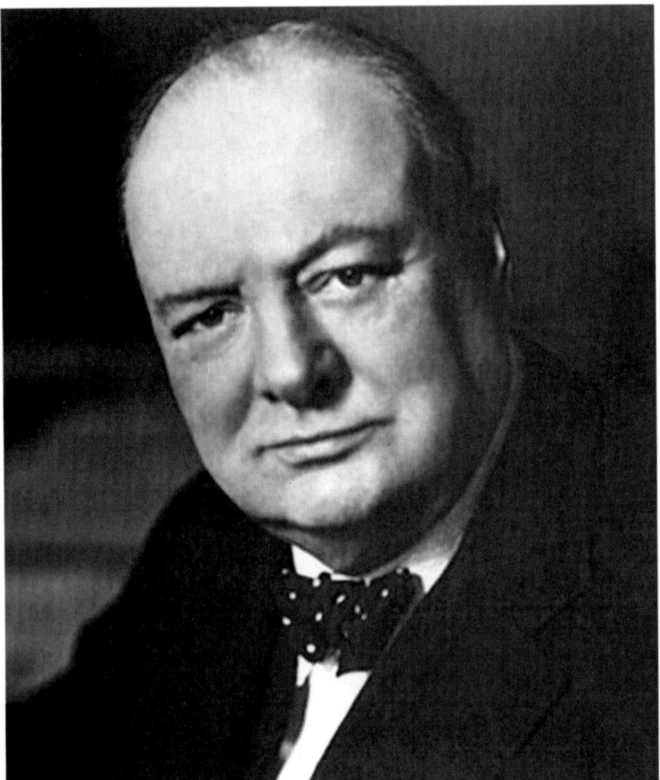

Winston Churchill

Having escaped a prison camp, beaten the Nazis, and been twice elected British Prime Minister, Winston Churchill is a singular model of resilience. Yet he was recurrently plagued by depression, or what he called his "black dog."

Some historians have suggested Churchill's depression originated with parental neglect. He was known to be deeply distressed by political failures, as he was following the disastrous assault on Istanbul in 1915. "I thought he would die of grief," his wife later said. In the aftermath, Churchill recovered his self-respect and confidence when his sister-in-law introduced him to watercolor painting.

Inspirational, In Spite of Depression

Great thinkers, artists, leaders, and explorers alike who have inspired us, even in the face of severe depression.

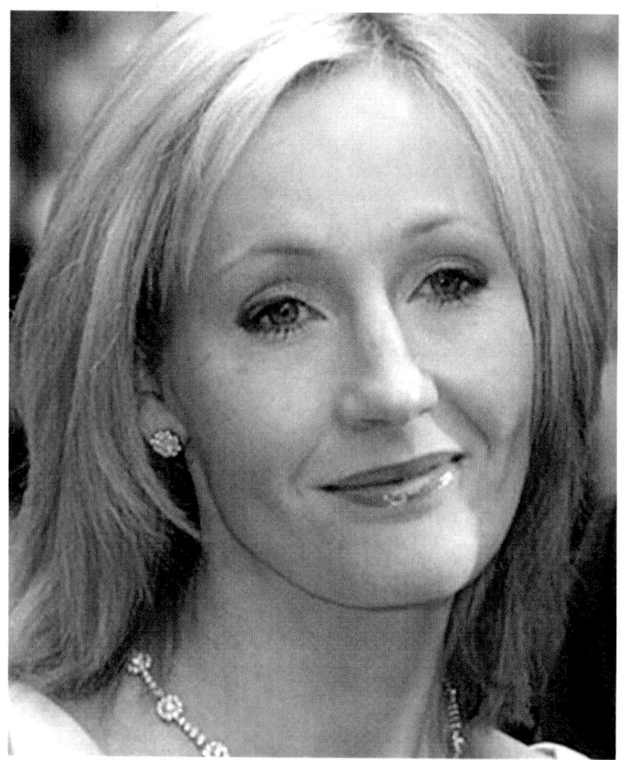

J.K. Rowling

The world would never have met Harry Potter if depression had gripped author J.K. Rowling any tighter than it did in the winter of 1993-94. The author-to-be was in her late twenties when she was diagnosed with clinical depression following a separation from the man she'd married a year prior.

Rowling has said she was nearly suicidal, and credits her recovery to a helpful doctor and love for her baby daughter. The newly single mom went on to pen most of *Harry Potter and the Philosopher's Stone* while her child slept in a nearby stroller.

Inspirational, In Spite of Depression

Great thinkers, artists, leaders, and explorers alike who have inspired us, even in the face of severe depression.

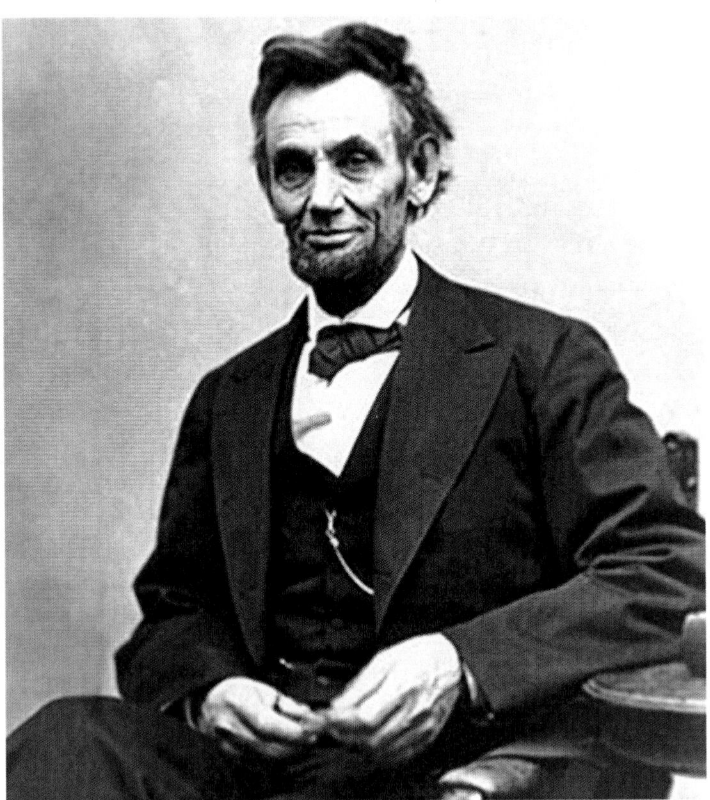

Abraham Lincoln

Depression didn't exist as a diagnosis in Lincoln's time, but there is no mistaking the symptoms that plagued the sixteenth president. Personal memories from those who knew Lincoln paint a picture of a profoundly despairing soul. He spoke of suicide even as a youth, quoted dark poems, wept openly, and often appeared lost in troubling thoughts. In the midst of one breakdown, he wrote to his law partner, "I am the most miserable man living. If what I feel were equally distributed to the whole human family, there would not be one cheerful face on the earth."

Lincoln did not so much emerge from his melancholy as put it to work. Keenly aware of the pain he'd endured, Lincoln knew he possessed tools for coping. He managed to communicate to a young America the value of clinging doggedly to a hopeful vision.

One of the things that helped Lincoln was his humor. One day, he asked a man who was sitting in his office, "How many legs does a dog have?" The man responded, "Four." Abe retorted, "But what if we say his tail is a leg, now how many legs does a dog have?" The man replied, "Well, he has five." Abe replied, "No, he only has four; just because we call his tail a leg doesn't make it a leg."

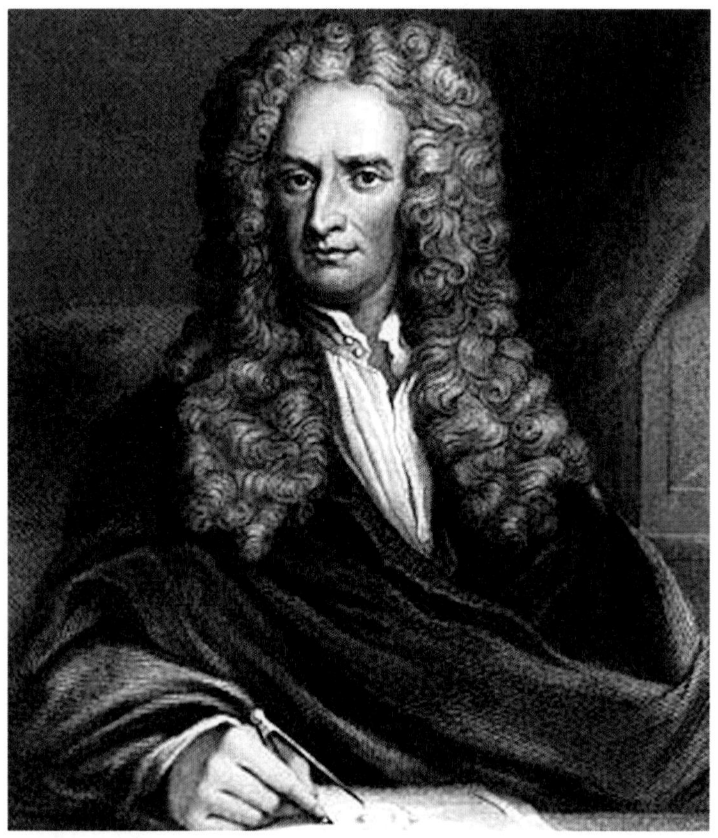

Isaac Newton

Isaac Newton did more to shape our understanding of the natural world than any other figure in history. His work is all the more remarkable considering the enormous psychological hurdles he overcame. Newtown was born prematurely, and probably illegitimately, into a broken family. His mother deserted him when he was three, leaving him to be raised by his elderly grandparents. As a teenager, he was riddled with guilt, as if his mother had left him behind as punishment for something he'd done. Newton has been characterized by biographers as neurotic, obsessive, hypochondriacal, detached, and prone to self-inflicted injury.

Inspirational, In Spite of Depression

Great thinkers, artists, leaders, and explorers alike who have inspired us, even in the face of severe depression.

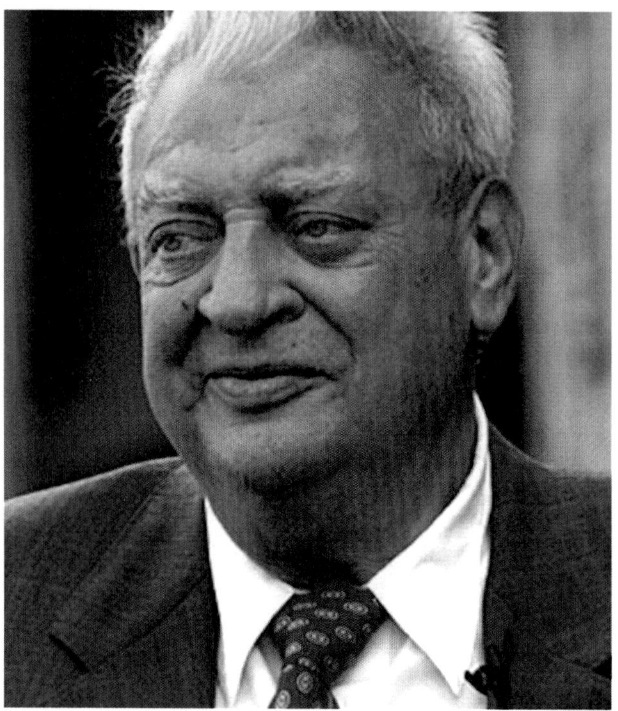

Rodney Dangerfield

Many comedians trade on their own misery. Dangerfield, a comic's comic, was at no loss for material. Rodney traced his depression back to an unhappy childhood, when he was abandoned by his father and raised by a mother he described as overbearing and cold. From a legitimately sad and lonely life, Rodney spun sad-sack schtick. But even when the laughs came—and with them, the audiences and the money—Dangerfield continued to struggle with clinical depression.

Before launching into a string of self-deprecating one liners, Rodney used to preface, "Nothing goes right for me." He may have been unable to see his life any other way, but he did earn plenty of respect from fans and fellow comics.

Inspirational, In Spite of Depression

Great thinkers, artists, leaders, and explorers alike who have inspired us, even in the face of severe depression.

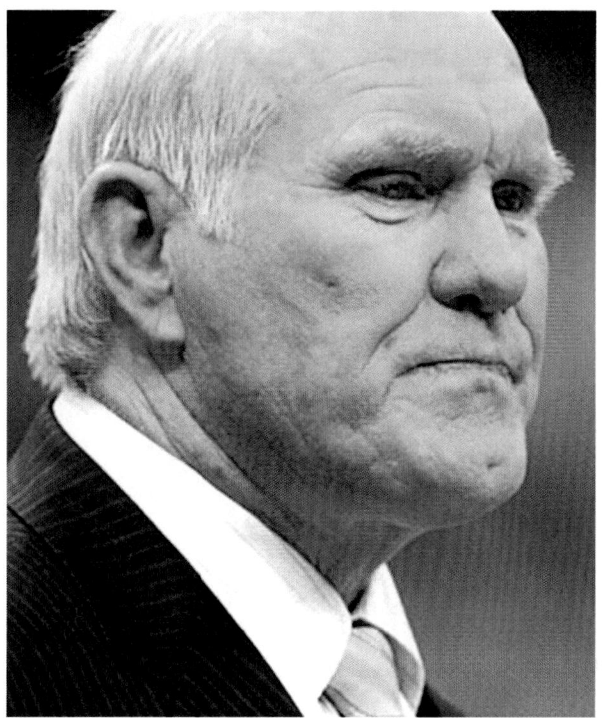

Terry Bradshaw

If ever there were evidence that depression is not a byproduct of weakness, Terry Bradshaw is it. The 6'3," 215 lb. NFL star has spoken with characteristic frankness about surviving the depression, pain, and adversity in his life. He's also known for his high-spirited, good-old-boy personality as a sports announcer, providing a lesson in how adroitly depressives can hide their condition. Bradshaw's enviable career titles have included Super Bowl MVP (twice), Hall of Famer, actor, Emmy-winning sportscaster, best-selling author, recording artist, and motivational speaker. Long after hanging up his #12 jersey for the Pittsburgh Steelers, Bradshaw is a genuine inspiration.

Inspirational, In Spite of Depression

Great thinkers, artists, leaders, and explorers alike who have inspired us, even in the face of severe depression.

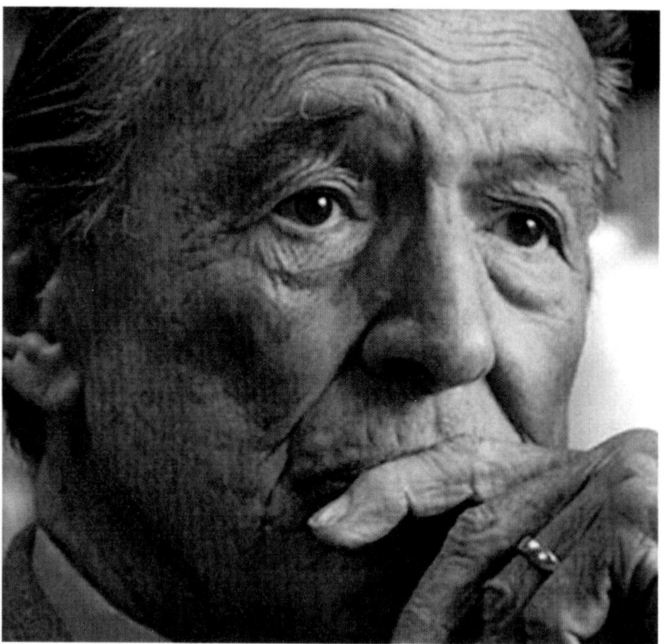

Mike Wallace

It took nearly twenty years for the revered *60 Minutes* anchor to publicly acknowledge his first bout with depression back in 1982. In the midst of a high-profile legal trial, Wallace was overcome with feelings of hopelessness and attempted suicide by sleeping-pill overdose. He was saved when his wife called for help.

Wallace's family doctor initially had told him to "forget about the word 'depression'" since there was so much stigma attached. "In retrospect, what a damn fool he was," Wallace told PBS. "There's nothing to be ashamed of about depression." The news veteran found his way up and out of with a combination of talk therapy and medication. Though the condition recurred—once after a broken wrist and again after turning seventy-five—Wallace knew by then that depression could be managed and was able to recover again.

Inspirational, In Spite of Depression

Great thinkers, artists, leaders, and explorers alike who have inspired us, even in the face of severe depression.

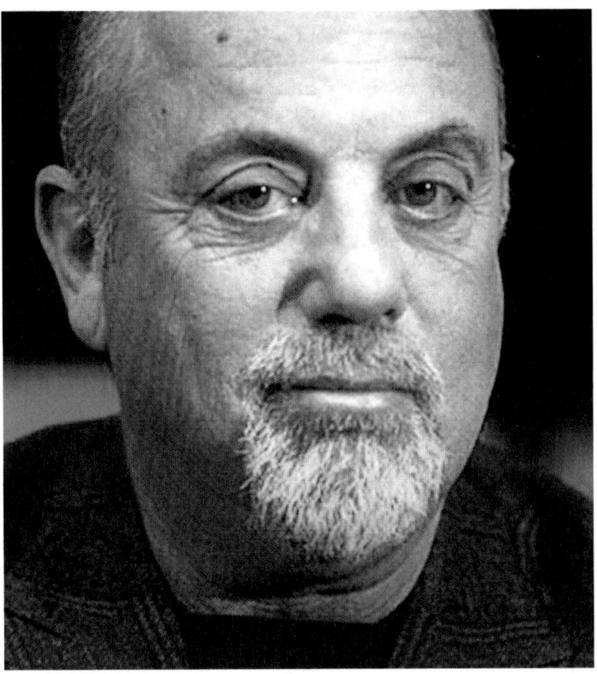

Billy Joel

He has millions of fans, millions of dollars, and his songs have been played millions of times around the world, but the Piano Man still does battle with his dark side. In 1970, when he was broke and sleeping in Laundromats to stay warm, Joel made a suicide attempt by drinking a bottle of furniture polish. He subsequently checked himself into a psych ward, and after living with the other patients, he said he was permanently cured of self-pity. The songwriter's suicide note inspired the lyrics for "Tomorrow is Today" from his debut record, and he later wrote the upbeat "You're Only Human (Second Wind)" as a message to teens contemplating suicide.

Inspirational, In Spite of Depression

Great thinkers, artists, leaders, and explorers alike who have inspired us, even in the face of severe depression.

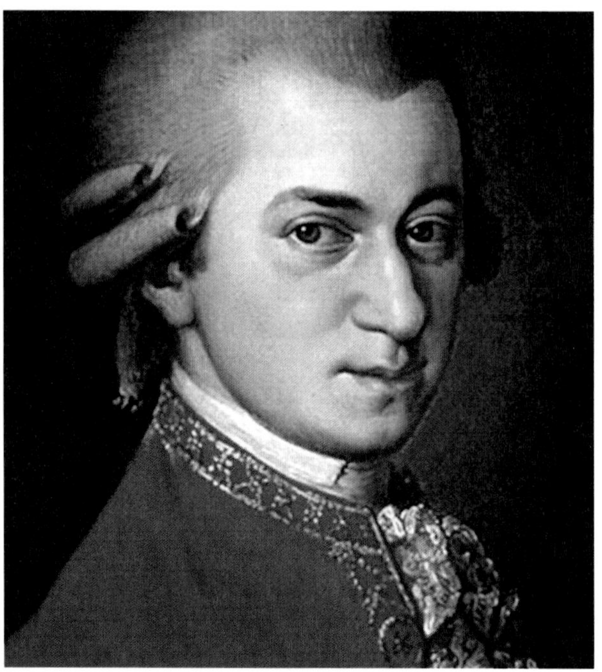

Mozart

"If people could see into my heart, I should almost feel ashamed. To me everything is cold—cold as ice."

These words are from a 1790 letter between Mozart and a friend from whom he sought sympathy (and money). They're particularly striking for a true genius whose music has brightened and comforted so many.

The great composer knew sadness and loss nearly all of his life, beginning in his youngest years when his talent was exploited for his family's financial and social gain. Even at the height of his fame, Mozart lived on the edge of ruin and despair. Late in his short life, he became "ill and consumed by worries and anxieties" which often left him sleepless. But in the year before he died, Mozart was prolific. His final compositions, including "The Magic Flute," are among his most triumphant.

Inspirational, In Spite of Depression

Great thinkers, artists, leaders, and explorers alike who have inspired us, even in the face of severe depression.

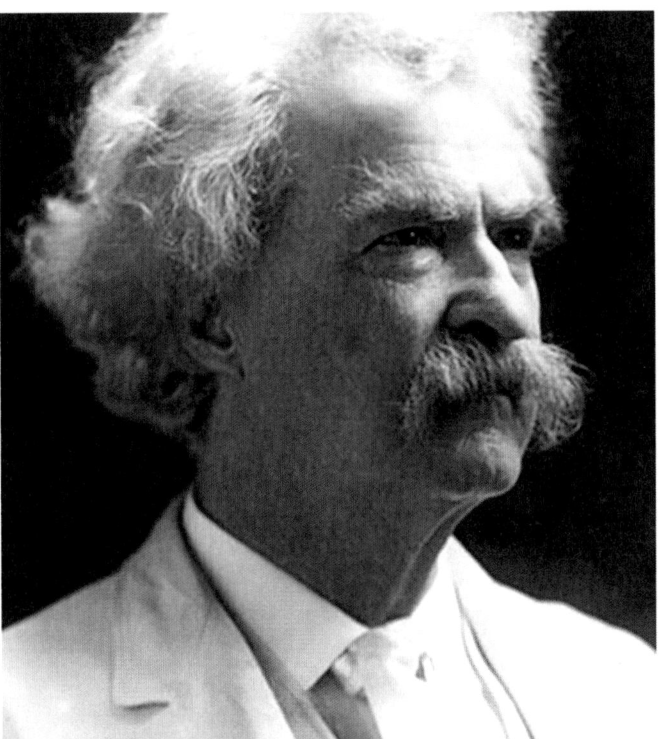

Mark Twain

By his own admission, Mark Twain's autobiographical accounts are part fiction. Colorful, ribald, and funny as heck, Twain's writing is more closely identified with cheerfully avoiding life's hardships rather than being overcome by them. But biographical researchers have identified a significant thread of depression in the author's life, most notably in his last fifteen years when he lost his wife, two daughters, and a close friend. "Everyone is a moon," he wrote in 1897's *Following the Equator*, "and has a dark side which he never shows to anybody."

Better, though, to leave you with another great quote from the American novelist:

"Twenty years from now, you will be more disappointed by the things you didn't do than by the ones you did. So throw off the bowlines. Sail away from the safe harbor. Catch the trade winds in your sails. Explore. Dream. Discover."

Sometimes, at least in your mind, kick off the pressures of life by following these next five precious gems:

Work like you don't need the money

Love like nobody has hurt you.

Dance like nobody is watching.

Sing like nobody is listening.

Live as if this was paradise on earth.

I've always been a dreamer as far back as I can remember, which is about the age of three or four. At that time, our family was living in Hot Springs, Arkansas, a small town nestled in Hot Springs National Park. We moved there in 1954 where my father opened a health food store called "Foods for Health."

I remember when my dad got through with the cash register tape, I would ask him for it and I would roll it all out and reroll it and write jokes and draw pictures on the register tape and stand outside and as people passed by, I would ask them if they wanted to buy a joke for a nickel; and to my surprise some did.

It's good to dream. I love Martin Luther King Junior's famous statement, "I have a dream." If you have a dream in your heart, it will inspire you in a way nothing else can. My first name is Hampton, which was given to me by my biological parents and when I was adopted, my new parents kept all our first names and changed our middle and, of course, last names. My older brothers are Bill, John, and Bob. My grandfather's first name was Hampton and my father's first name was Hampton, so I imagine they said, "why not, we'll call him Hampton.

People tell me, "That's such a unique name. I like it." I think they say that because they cannot think of anything else to say about a first name like Hampton; it's kind of like "a boy named Sue."

But as I got older, and into my adult life, I would dream about becoming rich. How? Well, the chain of motels, the Hampton Inn's, I would dream, actually day dream, that one day a limousine would pull up in front of my house and two men would come to my front door. We would open the door and they would say, "We are attorneys at law with the law firm of money, money, and more money? Is your biological name Hampton James Johnson the Third? And after I said "It is," then they would say, "We represent the late Hampton James Johnson the Second's estate. Your biological father is the owner of the chain of Hampton Inn Motels and you are the sole surviving heir and he has left you everything."

You might be thinking that's absurd, but that dream got me through many difficult and sometimes despondent times in my life. Whatever you think on, think on good things, this will actually strengthen your mental and spiritual immune system. We actually have three immune systems. The first is our physical immune system; exercise and eating the right foods strengthens this immune system. The second is our mental or psychological immune system. We can strengthen this immune system by reading good things and memorizing. If you want to ward off Alzheimer's and dementia, spend time memorizing; this strengthens and expands the mind. Get away from television. For the most part, it makes mush out of our minds. Your neuropathways in the mind actually atrophy when you watch a lot of television. Television and movies remove your ability of creativity and the desire to dream and oftentimes leave you depressed.

The third immune system is our spiritual immune system. We strength our spiritual immune system by spending time getting to know our Creator, through helping others, by not settling for mediocrity, striving for excellence in every facet of our lives, reading the Bible and meditating upon what we have read, by praying and finally spending time in nature by taking in all the beauty around us with a thankful heart.

I just found an article on the internet on how *television* can actually shorten your life span.

> Study: An hour of TV can shorten your life by 22 minutes.
>
> After the age of 25, watching 60 minutes of television is like smoking two cigarettes, researchers find.

Watching an hour of TV after the age of 25 can shorten the viewer's life by just under 22 minutes, according to researchers in Australia.

The AFP news agency said scientists at the School of Population Health at the University of Queensland studied 11,000 Australian adults who were aged at least 25 in the year 2000.

The academics checked their data against an estimate from 2008 that Australians aged 25 or above watched TV for 9.8 billion hours.

This was associated with the loss of 286,000 years of life, the AFP said.

An extrapolation of these figures found that a single hour of TV was responsible for the loss of just under 22 minutes of life, the news agency reported.

Smoking two cigarettes has approximately the same effect.

The problem is not actually TV itself but the lack of activity by the viewer for long periods, the researches said. Cardiovascular disease, diabetes, excess weight and other health problems are associated with a sedentary lifestyle.

Population Implications

Lennert Veerman, who was involved in the study, said the research showed watching television was "in the same ballpark as smoking and obesity," according to a report in The Guardian newspaper.

"While smoking rates are declining, watching TV is not, which has implications at a population level," he said according to the report.

A previous study in Australia found there was an 8 percent greater risk of dying prematurely associated with watching an hour of TV a day.

"We've taken that study and translated it into what it means for life expectancy in Australia given how much TV we watch," Veerman said.

The latest research was published in the British Journal of Sports Medicine.

Story: 15 minutes of fitness a day can add 3 years to your life.

Meanwhile, a large study in Taiwan found that doing just 15 minutes of moderate exercise a day might add three years to your life.

Lead researcher Chi Pang Wen of Taiwan's National Health Research Institutes said dedicating 15 minutes a day to a moderate form of exercise, like brisk walking, would benefit anyone.

"It's for men, women, the young and old, smokers, healthy and unhealthy people. Doctors, when they see any type of patient, this is a one-size-fits-all type of advice," Wen told Reuters in a telephone interview.

Wen and colleagues, who published their findings in medical journal The Lancet on Tuesday, tracked over 416,000 participants for 13 years, analyzing their health records and reported levels of physical activity each year.

I might add to this study that I read the comments of one critic about the above study that said reading a book may do the same, based upon the fact that you're just sitting usually when you're reading or lying down which equates to no physical activity; but, at

least while you're reading, you are exercising and stimulating your mental immune system.

I'll guarantee you, the makers of movies are dreamers and they have taken their dreams and put them into films and have made millions doing it; so instead watching of an exciting movie, why not make one or live one out in your life.

6 ways Hollywood lies to us about the workplace
By Sonia Acosta, CareerBuilder Writer

The ever-popular HBO series "Sex and the City" is rarely thought of as a workplace show, but if we take a closer look, we can see it is riddled with workplace clichés.
Bing: Worst movie bosses

Carrie Bradshaw, our main gal, somehow makes an extravagant living from one weekly newspaper column she often writes in her underwear while smoking what seems to be a smokeless cigarette inside her New York City apartment. Miranda Hobbes, a "busy" corporate lawyer never seems too busy for lunches, parties, shopping or long walks around the city with best pal Carrie. Charlotte York is a museum curator who rarely curates anything but her obsession with finding Mr. Right and having Mr. Right Jr. Finally, but certainly not least in any sense of the word, Samantha Jones is a successful public relations practitioner despite a reputation the size of New York City itself. How ironic.

Recently, over on the humor website, Cracked.com, one writer was fed up with the annoying clichés about women that keep popping up in movies. Tired of seeing gorgeous actresses playing the supposedly unattractive sister and an unrealistic emphasis on the glories of shopping, Christina H. penned "6 obnoxious assumptions

Hollywood makes about women." The list is not only funny but also accurate if you stop and think about how many movies these annoying tropes occur in. It also got us thinking that Hollywood's not just inaccurately portraying women in movies or on TV — its off the mark about what it's like for the average worker in today's economy.

As a result, we bring you six ways Hollywood lies to us about the workplace...

1. All the beautiful people

Ever notice all the long-legged, luscious-haired, model-types walking around your office? What about all of the strapping, buff and impeccably-dressed men? We didn't think so.

Hollywood can often make it seem like unattractive, overweight or simple-humored people don't work. Skills? Who needs 'em, right? As long as you look good and utter funny, clever remarks all day, you're bound to grow business and make bushels of money.

Sure statistics exist regarding attractive people getting hired over, promoted instead of or paid more than unattractive ones, but these people also have skills, education or the ability to move business in some significant way. A pretty face might help, but if that's all you got, it's not going to cut it in the real world.

Hollywood examples: "The In Crowd", "Confessions of a Shopaholic"," Grey's Anatomy"

2. Executives work? Nah...

The recent Sarah Jessica Parker movie "I Don't Know How She Does It" in which she plays the role of an international fund manager, wife and mother, portrays an unrealistic schedule for such an executive-level job.

Christina Gombar, author of fiction, memoir and literary criticism says, "No way, no way, no way, would an international fund manager get into work at 9:00 a.m. She would be working around the clock with her terminal from home. She wouldn't have time to shoot snarky emails to her female work mates. My pals who are traders can't talk to me on the phone and can only send the shortest texts."

Beverly Solomon, a marketer, creative director and author based in Austin, Texas believes Hollywood portrays executives and entrepreneurs as "rich, uncaring crooks who made their fortunes by stepping on the regular people."

Solomon, having worked for Diane Von Furstenberg and Ralph Lauren, looks down on this cliché, noting "both were great entrepreneurs who built their businesses with vision and tenacity, and are good people."

Hollywood examples: "You've Got Mail", "Be Kind Rewind", "Wall Street"

3. Your outfit? Anything goes!

A suit? Slacks? Minimal cleavage? That's crazy talk. According to Hollywood, club wear is quite suitable for the workplace, and even welcome. How else do you plan to get that big promotion or spark up that all-appropriate office romance?

Christina McCale, marketing academic, career coach and co-editor of "Start Your Internet Business: 36 Things You Need to Know" says, "While Millennials are changing a lot of things about the way we dress in the workplace, the reality is there is still a level of professionalism expected, and usually, that isn't reflected in 'Britney-esque' outfits."

McCale cautions you should always remember who your boss is. "They're not likely to appreciate you wearing club wear to the office meeting. And even more likely — they won't take you seriously."

Hollywood examples: "My Boss's Daughter", "View from the Top", "Legally Blonde"

4. Work is so easy.

"The common [so-called 'webpreneurial'] storyline on TV shows or movies goes like this: person gets idea; they set up a website; next day money is rolling in," says McCale. Citing another unrealistic example, she adds, "Crime scene investigators strategically hold up flashlights; miraculously evidence appears. The reality is CSIs across the country aren't exactly running around in Louis Vuitton shoes. CSI work is hard, and many crime labs are not nearly as well equipped as the ones you see on TV."

On TV and in movies, people make more witty remarks than they complete important projects. They hang out all day, barely ever sitting at a computer or on a phone call. Pranks are a regular part of the work day, and talking to the boss in the same way you talk to your poker buddies is acceptable. In today's economy, it's hard to imagine anyone's workday is that carefree.

Hollywood examples: "The Office", "30 Rock", "Clerks", "Will & Grace"

5. Money is no object.

Wouldn't it be nice to live in a movie or TV sitcoms where you can be an out of work actor, waitress or writer and still live in a lavish New York

City apartment, buy $500 Louis Vuittons, sip on warm delights in a coffee shop all day, and barely ever go to work? TV shows like “Friends” and “Sex and the City,” and characters like Rachel Green, Joey Tribbiani and Carrie Bradshaw give us the false hope that we can actually work little and live a lot. In a post-recession economy, many workers are deciding how often they can afford to buy coffee each week, but you don’t see that on TV.

Hollywood examples: “The 40 Year Old Virgin“, “Cheers“, “The Real Housewives [of any city]”, “Modern Family“

6. Your boss is a horrible person and/or an idiot.

You’ve probably had a boss that wasn’t the brightest bulb or even the nicest person you’ve ever met, but he or she wasn’t necessarily worthless. In fact, unless you’ve had an unfortunate run of luck, your bosses probably ranged from OK people to great leaders. Your average Hollywood bosses, however, either exist to make your life miserable with outrageous demands and endless piles of work, or they’re incompetent fools who can barely tie their own shoes much less manage a team.

“While there are always going to be bosses who are ‘clueless’ [it’s] not a good idea to point that out to them,” says McCale. “Worse, don’t make how you ‘feel they are clueless’ obvious in front of others.”

Hollywood examples: “The Devil Wears Prada“, “Horrible Bosses“, “Nine to Five“

Why it matters

“The shame is, many teens and 20-somethings base career choices on what they see on TV, and TV just isn’t a great career counselor, because shows aren't meant to do that," says McCale. " TV and movies are entertainment. They are geared for a shorter attention span, and to use elements of truth to propel a storyline forward."

While work can be fun, and some companies might have a more informal working environment than others, you might not want to model your workplace behavior after what you see on TV and in movies.

Sonia Acosta is a writer and blogger for CareerBuilder.com and its job blog, The Work Buzz. She researches and writes about job search strategy, career management, hiring trends and workplace issues.

Bottom of Form

Make no mistake, television networks and movie makers want to make money and a lot of it. If the public-that's you and I-are watching the garbage that they are throwing at us, then they are going to keep getting more immoral, more vulgar until there are no morals in our society and few people will be able to distinguish right from wrong, especially our children.

Hollywood definitely has an agenda when it comes to the writers of sitcoms and movies. I just went to dictionary.com and pulled this definition for sitcom: "a situation comedy as found on television. These sitcoms are made for juvenile minds." That makes sense; because that is about the level of immaturity and intelligence that you find in a sitcom today. I also pulled a definition for immature from dictionary.com: "emotionally undeveloped; juvenile; childish."

Overtime, I have collected some quotes that have helped me through some tough times. Check these out:

√ "When life gives you scraps make quilts."
√ "Desperate times call for desperate measures."
√ "No matter how far you have gone on the wrong road, turn back."

- √ "Turn your face to the sun and the shadows fall behind you."
- √ "You can outdistance that which is running after you, but not what is running inside you."
- √ "Faith is like a bird that feels dawn breaking and sings while it is still dark."
- √ "Act as though it is impossible to fail."
- √ "A smooth sea never made a skillful mariner."
- √ "If you get up one more time than you fall, you will make it through."
- √ "A person is just as big as the thing that makes him angry."
- √ "Anger is only one letter short of danger."
- √ "A healthy attitude is contagious, but don't wait to catch it from others. Be a carrier."
- √ "May the road rise to meet you. May the wind be always at your back. May the sun shine warm upon your face, and the rain fall soft upon your fields; and until we meet again, may God hold you in the palm of His hand "Change your thoughts and you change your world."

The answer to depression is not chronic ingestion of medications or drugs. At times, there may be a need to place a patient on an antidepressant for a short time, but to leave him or her on an antidepressant indefinitely is wrong, unethical, and demonstrates an indifference to a patient's real need, and can be a form of medical malpractice.

Exercise is where every person needs to start when faced with functional or non-functional depression. There are really three areas to fitness or exercise:

- Cardiovascular exercise
- Strength training
- Flexibility (This is really the third pillar of fitness.)

"Flexibility is the third pillar of fitness, next to cardiovascular conditioning and strength training," says David Geier, the director of sports medicine at the Medical University of South Carolina, in Charleston. In fact, flexibility can help your body reach its optimum fitness level, may play a role in injury prevention, and even contribute to staving off conditions like arthritis and more serious illnesses.

Here's how it works: When you stretch a muscle, you lengthen the tendons, or muscle fibers, that attach it to the bone. "The longer these fibers are, the more you can increase the muscle in size when you do your strength training," says Geier.

That means that a more flexible muscle has the potential to become a stronger muscle, too. In turn, building strong muscle fibers may boost your metabolism and your fitness level.

Flexible muscles also make everyday activities easier on your body and may decrease your risk of certain injuries. Common behaviors, like hunching over the computer, can shorten some muscles. That, along with the natural loss of muscle elasticity that occurs with aging, can set you up so any quick or awkward motion (lunging to catch a glass before it teeters off the table, for example) could stretch your muscles beyond their limit, resulting in a strain or a tear. "Even if you're aerobically fit, it helps to be limber, too, so your body can easily adapt to physical stressors," says Margot Miller, a physical therapist in Duluth, Minnesota, and a spokesperson for the American Physical Therapy association.

What's more, stretching may improve your circulation, increasing blood flow to your muscles. Having good circulation can help protect you against a host of illnesses, from diabetes to kidney disease. Greater flexibility has even been linked to a lower risk of cardiovascular disease.

How much stretching do we need? To increase your flexibility, start with about ten minutes of stretching a day, focusing on the major muscle groups: upper body (arms, shoulders, neck), back, and lower body (thighs, calves, ankles). Then, depending on how you typically spend your time, focus on specific stretches for problem-prone areas. So, if you're pretty much parked at a desk from nine to five, you'll want to give extra attention to your lower back and shoulders. If you're on the move—picking up toddlers and bags of groceries, perhaps—concentrate on your hamstrings and arms.

If you don't have ten minutes a day to spare, stretching just a few times a week can be nearly as beneficial. In fact, that may be enough to help you stay supple once you've gotten there. A study published in the Journal of Strength Conditioning and Research found that after stretching every day for a month, participants who went on to stretch just two or three times a week maintained their degree of flexibility. Those who stopped stretching, however, lost about 7 percent of their hip range of motion within a month.

"The more you do it, the more you will get out of it—both physically and psychologically," says Geier.

I remember watching Michael Jordan playing basketball years ago. Sometimes, he would start the game with some type of injury to his ankle where the commentators said Michael probably wouldn't play at all that night; but inevitably his coach Phil Jackson would have him play a little. And someone said before the game began that Phil Jackson wanted to keep Michael Jordan's muscles, ligaments, and tendons around the injured ankle limber, so his ankle wouldn't get stiff.

Stretching also helps bring in fresh blood to the injured area and remove injured blood cells and tissue. More blood, more oxygen, more white blood cells, bring quicker healing.

I want to interject something right here about healing. If you smoke and you have an injury, especially an open wound injury, healing will be reduced by 80 percent, especially if you are diabetic and you smoke. The single greatest thing you can do for your health, if you smoke, is to stop smoking right now. If you just read this and you smoke, get up, gather all your tobacco paraphernalia, your cigarettes, cigars, or chewing tobacco and take and throw them into the trashcan now. You can do it cold turkey. I know it can be done. I did it. And if I did it, anyone can.

When I opened up to the internet today, I clicked on an NBC video of Michael Douglas on the David Letterman show announcing for the first time to the world, to all of us who have loved his acting that he has Stage 4 throat cancer and that he is presently going through chemotherapy and radiation treatment. One doctor said because it is stage 4, sometimes they have success rates of up to 80 percent. The doctor also said it is the size of a walnut located at the base of his tongue.

But the reason that I even bring this up is for what Michael Douglas said, which will remain in the halls of my memory for a long time, and I hope it does for you, too. He said of his cancer that it was his lifestyle of drinking and smoking that caused his cancer. Alcohol changes the cellular structure of the cells in the throat, which then makes it easier for all the carcinogens in tobacco to bring on cancer.

I'm saddened indeed for Michael Douglas and for his lovely wife of this news. He continues to lose weight and will continue to as the physicians administer chemotherapy and radiation; but I was very encouraged to see and hear his upbeat attitude. We can soar like eagles with the right attitude.

Alcohol, tobacco, and coffee are three of the worst things you can become addicted to. Alcohol kills more people than just about everything else combined; tobacco will kill the rest.

Today, I talked with a patient who was going into the endoscopy lab for an EGD and colonoscopy. He was a male, fifty-one years of age. I was going down through my list of questions I routinely ask my patients and when I asked him if he experiences any gastric reflux, he said he did. Then he went on to tell me how coffee causes gastric reflux. I told him you are absolutely correct. I asked how much coffee he has been consuming a day and he said upwards to four thirty-two-ounce jugs a day; that is sixteen cups of coffee a day. How would you have time to do anything else?

Coffee will actually permanently impair or permanently damage the cardiac sphincter (LES), the door that allows food and drink to enter your stomach from your esophagus. When that occurs, acid and gases will reflux or regurgitate back up the esophagus and now that acid and those gases will enter the trachea and into the lungs, into the sinuses through the nose and inflame the tender lining of the esophagus and the lungs.

Very hot drinks and very cold drinks can also change the cellular structure of the cells that line our oral pharynx, esophagus, and stomach.

The Japanese have a very high incidence of stomach and throat cancers. They consume very hot drinks; and very hot or very cold drinks taken in for a long time will eventually change the cellular structure of the cells and set you up for cancer.

I know someone who has MS (Multiple Sclerosis). She is constantly drinking ice water or cold soft drinks. This isn't helping her MS and it certainly isn't doing her esophagus and stomach any good. She complains of being hot all the time and states that her MS makes her feel hot and she is just trying to stay cool. But this is a myth. Ice cold drinks don't actually cool you down—they heat you up. Your brain senses this sudden change in temperature of your body as if you were in the freezing cold of winter and therefore it begins to bring the blood to your body surface to heat you up. So your mind sends a signal to your hypothalamus (the temperature regulating center in the brain) and you begin to feel hot again. So you drink more ice cold drinks and your hypothalamus sends more signals and you heat up again. And so this vicious cycle continues cold and hot, cold and hot until in some cases you become totally exhausted and your body just wears out.

Just this weekend, I was invited to have dinner with some friends and one of the couples that were there I have known for over twenty years. He is retired now at the age of sixty-two. But for the last two to three years, he has been plagued with an irritating cough, which some of the physicians have diagnosed as bronchitis. He turns his head every now and then to cough. At times, I can see he needs more air. He doesn't smoke and I don't think he ever has. He has had all kinds of tests done and they haven't come up with anything conclusive that he or his doctors can get their arms around.

He asked me, "You have any ideas of what to do?" He is at his wits end and, quite frankly, isn't enjoying life to its fullest as he should be. I shared with him some things I believe will help him.

Each morning when you get up go to the kitchen and drink two big glasses of water at least eight ounces—I prefer about sixteen ounces, but whatever you're comfortable with—make one of the glasses hot but not coffee hot and definitely not just lukewarm; that tastes awful. Do not drink ice water or any ice drinks of any kind, especially soda pops. The most common scenario you will find in a fast food restaurant, when you see people eating for example is: a hamburger, French-fries, and soft drink. And if you observe closely, you will see most people only chew each bite just a few times and then they wash the partially chewed food down with whatever they are drinking. The stomach and intestines now become chilled, which slows digestion in the stomach and slows or even stops peristalsis in the small intestine.

Peristalsis is the progressive wave of contraction and relaxation of a tubular *muscular system*, especially *the* alimentary canal, by which the contents are forced through the system. So now, your body has to ratchet up the temperature inside your body so digestion can move along; this is one of the reasons people complain of being hot when they drink ice cold drinks, whether the liquid is soda pop, beer, or water.

When you don't chew your food thoroughly enough by washing it down with some kind of drink, even water, your body's response is to secrete more acid because that food must be broken down before it moves into the small intestine. Why? In the small intestine, what you need to sustain health is absorbed or taken up into the bloodstream from where it is distributed to the billions of cells in your body. Your body can't take up small chunks of food into the blood stream. Not only is your stomach churning out more acid, your stomach isn't getting much rest before the next meal.

Soda pop manufacturers know all this and the number one thing they want you to do is to buy more soda pop. To accomplish this, they put lots of sugar, about ten teaspoons for each eight-ounce of soda and lots of sodium and of course as much caffeine as is allowed by law and many other substances. They don't really ever want your thirst quenched.

Here is something right out of Wikipedia off the internet—Coca-Cola:

> The Pure Food and Drug Act was initially concerned with ensuring products were labeled correctly. Later efforts were made to outlaw certain products that were not safe, followed by efforts to outlaw products that were safe but not effective. For example, an attempt to outlaw Coca-Cola in 1909 because of its excessive caffeine; caffeine re-

> placed cocaine as the active ingredient in coca-cola in 1903. In the case *United States v. Forty Barrels and Twenty Kegs of Coca-Cola*, the judge found that Coca-Cola had a right to use caffeine as it saw fit, although excessive litigation costs caused Coca-Cola to settle out of court with the United States Government. The caffeine amount was reduced.

The only drink that will really quench your thirst and not make your stomach hurt is cool water and if possible, spring-fed water; because after all, our bodies are 75 percent water—not 75 percent soda pop, alcohol, or coffee. There is a difference.

I then instructed him, "After you finish showering but before you get out of the shower, turn up the heat as far as is comfortable and do a slow 360 turn and then turn down the temperature as cold as is comfortable and do a 360 turn then increase the temperature again and now let the cold water fall upon your face and chest. Repeat that routine three times and finish with water that returns your body to the ambient temperature of the room."

When you turn the water to cold, that will open up those little dependent airway passages deep down in your lungs and it will often cause you to cough, cleaning your lungs. The cold water also constricts your blood vessels, especially in your sinuses. What this will do is open up your sinuses and allow you to breath freely again; this is the reaction you have when you take nasal decongestant medications, but without the nasty side effects. It's actually an exhilarating experience.

When you finish your shower, dry off using a brisk friction rub with your towel all over your body. This really gets the circulation going throughout your body. This also will raise your white blood cell count. Then go outside and do some deep breathing; slowly inhale through your nose and slowly exhale through your mouth. If you have time, do your deep breathing exercises while you walk.

Every day, I work with people who come to work and are suffering with some type of nasal congestion. When I ask if they are feeling okay, they typically tell me "It's allergies." Environmental allergies do play a big role in all our lives but, oftentimes, that's not the real cause of our nasal congestion.

Just the other day, I heard a doctor on one of these news channels answer the question of why children have so many allergies. He said it is primarily two-fold:

1. Children's allergies are related to all the vaccines and immunizations they are receiving.
2. Children's allergies also come from all the antibiotics they are receiving for conditions they should not be taking antibiotics.
3. I have heard reports that claim 60 percent of children's allergies are caused by dairy products.

We have become a nation so dependent upon medications and drugs that we need a drug to get us going in the morning; we need a drug to keep us going through the day; and we need a drug to get to sleep on, and this vicious cycle continues until our mind tells our bodies, "I'm checking out; I can't take this any longer," and many times, we collapse under the stress.

Fear is an emotion that millions of people struggle with every day of their lives." I wish the term inferiority complex had never been printed because then millions of people would not even know they had an inferiority complex," so writes Henry C. Link, Ph.D. over 60 years ago.

Has the grip of fear been loosened over the past 60 years? No!! More than ever people are living in fear-fear of the past, fear of the future and fear of the present.

Henry C. Link, Ph.D continues: "Most fears are actually generated by too much reading, thinking and talking. They do not, as a rule, just happen. We nurse them and feed them until, from an inconsequential trifle, they have grown to monstrous proportions. The mother who avidly reads the extensive literature on bringing up children becomes increasingly fearful of how to deal with them and well she may. The young woman too fussy about her appearance soon worries too much over what people will think of her. Groups of people who learnedly discuss the state of the country often turn pessimism into fear."

Henry C. Link, Ph.D goes on: "A young man told me that he could not sleep. He gave me a long psychological explanation of how this had come about. "Can you help me get rid of this obsession?" he asked. "No," was my reply. "Then what can I do?" he implored. "Run around the block at night until you are ready to drop. What you need is exertion. You have put too much of your physical energies into imagining things. If you run hard enough, you will automatically relax and go to sleep. You have thought yourself into this fear with your mind, you can run yourself out of it with your legs?"—and he did."

"A mother not long ago gave this significant summary of her life: "As a young woman I was troubled with many fears, one of which was the fear of insanity. After my marriage these fears still persisted. I started to worry, the baby would cry or the children would quarrel and I would have to straighten them out. Or I would suddenly remember that it was time to start dinner, or that the ironing had to be done. My fears about myself were being continually interrupted by family duties, and gradually they disappeared.

Now I look back on them with amusement."

I don't recommend having six children; but in our society we have smaller families and often too much leisure time on our hands which will kick the mind into high gear of meditating on old and new fears.

Remember when you learned how to dive. You stood on the side edge of the pool and placed your hands forward one on top the other out in front of your head and you leaned forward and then withdrew in fear. You tried it again with the same pose and again drew back in fear. With each hesitation your fears mounted. You stepped again to the edge of the pool, with good pose and this time everyone was counting, "one, two, three." And finally, you took the plunge and did a perfect belly flop and when you came out of the water all your friends were laughing. If, you had stopped trying to dive at this point your fears would have kept you from attempting to dive anymore. "If, however, you persisted, and continued to make awkward and painful dives, you finally went in smoothly and came up feeling pleased. You were on the way to becoming an expert."

"This is the basic psychology of overcoming fear and gaining confidence in every phase of life, and there is no escape from this process. Again and again we must plunge into the stream of life, adding one conquest to another, overcoming first this fear and then that. As Everson said, do the thing you fear and the death of fear is certain. Actually our fears are the forces that make us, when dealt with by decisive action, or that break us if dealt with by indecision, procrastination and ratiocination."

"Although generalizations are dangerous, I venture to say that at the bottom of most fears, both mild and severe, will be found an overactive mind and an underactive body. Hence, I have advised many people, in their quest for happiness, to use their heads less and their arms and legs more—-in useful work or play. We generate fears while we sit; we overcome them by action. Fear is nature's warning signal to get busy." Henry C. Link, Ph.D

A friend of mine called me recently and poured out his broken heart to me and I just want to share his text and I want to share my reply to him: "I have cried until I cannot cry anymore and then I have cried some more. I have screamed into the darkness of my soul asking the question why and I pray every night that I please not have to see tomorrows sunrise. I have never been so broken and hopeless. I would rather die than go through this and yet the pain just keeps growing. I don't want to live anymore. My candle has been blown out and I cry day and night. Where is God in all of this? I just don't know Hampton. Maybe I loved her too much and I had to lose her. I loved her with all that I had and I just don't understand how she could do this to me? I am trying hard to believe in the goodness of the Lord in the land of the living but I just don't know how I can hold on or even if I want to. She wants nothing to do with me except as it has to deal with the kids. I have worked my heart and soul out and all of the pieces are there to make this work but she refuses and only gets colder and colder. I don't want to see tomorrow Hampton-I really don't. I am tired of the pain and unending feelings of loss and despair..."

My response: "Hey friend-been praying for you. God loves you. Remember this will pass. Whatever happens-no matter what-you will come out a winner just don't ever give up. We love you."

Two days later I awoke at 1:25 a.m. and after tossing and turning I thought about my friend and sent this text message:

"—it is 2:20 a.m. eastern time and I am praying for you. The devil can't have you as long as I'm praying for you. Keep hanging on to Jesus. Don't let go. Someday you and I are going to ride Harleys together. Never give up. Jesus is coming. I love you brother but more importantly, God loves you with a Love I cannot."

The next morning I received another text from my friend: "Hampton I cannot tell you how much that means to me that you are praying for me at this hour and any time. I don't know what I am suppose to learn from this endless pain but I pray to God I learn it…my heart is SO broken and it is all I can do just to lift my head some days. I am tired of crying but the tears don't stop. Hampton she was the song in my heart and the fire in my soul and now it is all gone...I am a broken man! Thanks so much for your prayers Hampton and for your text. I can't even tell you where I am in life, I am so confused and hurt but I Know He holds the future…I just can't give up but it is sooo hard to hold on!

My response: "Thirty-one years ago I thought I wouldn't get my kids back from my ex-wife. I took a walk down a R/R track, fell down on my knees on those R/R tracks and wept and wept until I couldn't weep anymore and I finally just fell into the Great Loving arms of Jesus and I'm still there in His arms. Hang on-I need you man."

His last text to me: "Hampton I cry myself to sleep most nights and I thought I was in His loving arms. My mind tells me this truth but my heart has another truth. The sun is gently coming up on a new day that I do not want to see because it is just going to be filled with more of the same heartache I have known for another day to many! Maybe I loved her too much? I will keep holding on but I feel so black and dead on the inside. You are a good friend and I hope I learn the lesson, whatever it may be, so this pain won't be so endless and meaningless…"

The reason I'm sharing these texts with you is because as much as it hurt me to read my friends text and see how much he was hurting, it gave me peace and encouragement to know the few nanoseconds I took to communicate with him lifted his spirits. You'll be surprised how helping someone else will lift your spirits and make you forget about your problems.

I would be remiss if I didn't share some paragraphs from a book I bought at an antique shop in a little town of Sparta, Tennessee before closing this chapter on depression. The title is "Getting The Most Out Of Life". An Anthology from *The Reader's Digest.*

The chapter I want to share some things from is entitled "Why We All Have 'Ups and Downs'". This book was copyrighted in 1946, but the principles really haven't changed. "Dr. Rexford B Hersey of the University of Pennsylvania, who has been studying the rise and fall of human emotions for more than 17 years, has found that with all of us high and low spirits follow each other with a regularity almost as dependable as that of the tides. Outside circumstances merely advance or postpone slightly our regular periods of elation or depression. Instead of lifting you out of a slump, good news will give your spirits only a brief boost. And, conversely, bad news is less depressing when you're in an emotional "high." About 33 days after your particularly low or high spots, you're likely to find yourself feeling the same way again, for that is the normal length of the human "emotional cycle."

Wanting more information as to why our spirits go up and down and how we can use the constant ebb and flow of well-being more efficiently, Hersey made a detailed investigation of his own ups and downs.

In his low periods, he soon learned, he became more critical than at other times, and more irritable. He didn't want to be bothered by talking to people. He planned his schedule so that during his periods of depression he could devote himself to research, avoiding anything that required much self-confidence. During his high periods he scheduled his consultations and lectures.

He found that the work and output of his thyroid glands, his pituitary glands, his liver and other internal production plants varied markedly from week to week. The number of his red blood corpuscles, his blood cholesterol, each had —- as with all of us -— its own particular rhythm. The thyroid output, which to a greater extent than any other single factor determines the total "emotional cycle" rhythm, usually makes a round trip from low to high and back in from four to five weeks. Joining forces with Dr. Michael J. Bennett, endocrinologist of the Doctor's Hospital in Philadelphia, Hersey and Bennett decided, all the different factors work out to a "normal" cycle length of between 33 and 36 days.

Basically this emotional cycle consists of an over-all upbuilding and giving-out of energy. But the production and use of energy do not parallel each other quite evenly. First, we gradually build up more energy than we use. That makes us feel better and better, and we become more and more active and high-spirited. So we begin to use more energy than our system is producing. This keeps on until exhaustion of our surplus energy induces a reaction. We slump, often quite sharply, into feeling tired, depressed, discouraged.

We feel on top of the world for some time after our store of energy created for best conditions has begun to diminish. And conversely we feel low for some time after the rebuilding process has started up again. When everything seems hopeless we have already turned the corner.

There seems to be no difference in cycle length between men and women. With women, however, the results are confused by the menstrual cycle, which has its own ups and downs. When the emotional low of the menstrual cycle and the low of the basic emotional cycle coincide, an abnormally bad state of nervousness or anxiety may develop. Many unnecessary marital separations have unquestionable, Hersey and Bennett believe, been started at such a time.

You can see at once how tremendously important these findings can be to you personally. First of all, you can lessen any discouragement you may feel from temporary setbacks, any worry or anxiety about the future you experience when you are blue, by the realization that your depression may be a perfectly natural phase of living, soon to be followed by days or weeks of greater strength, assurance and optimism. No matter how dismal the outlook may seem to be, you simply won't be able to avoid feeling better presently."

Readers, we have been wonderfully and gloriously created and our loving Father has placed in us many ways to cope with everyday life even in a world gone amuck.

Don't settle for mediocrity in anything you do. Strive for excellence. Reach for the stars. Be the very best in whatever profession you are in.

I believe women as mothers have the highest calling of any human being ever born. Their role is more important than becoming President of the United States of America. The mother, most of the time, is responsible for molding the character of their children. That is an incredible responsibility; but one of the reasons we have such decadence in our society is because the mothers role has been belittled. It's one thing for men to become immoral, and I'm not diminishing their behavior, but when the women become like men in their immoral behavior, you have a society that is out of control and will end in social and economic ruin. That is "The Naked Truth."

Men, grass really isn't any greener on the other side of the fence. Someone once asked me why my wife and I don't wear wedding rings or for that matter any jewelry; does your church forbid that?

I responded, no. I guess because my parents never did-I don't.

"The men who have traveled most widely are those who have really seen what lies close about them at home." I don't know the author of this quote.

But what is amazing to me is that many of the people that have affairs or are having affairs now are wearing wedding bands. A wedding band will never keep you faithful to your wife or to your husband. That love has to be in the heart and guarded continuously.

I asked my mother, when I was younger why she and dad never wore a wedding band. My mother was born in 1913 and grew up on a large farm in the State of Michigan. She had two sisters and no brothers and so she learned how to harness a team and drive to town with it. But she said, "son, a wedding band is kind of like a yoke we use to put on oxen to keep them in the fence. That yoke worked to keep the oxen from sticking their heads between the barb wire strands-until-they got tired of eating the grass in their pasture or until they saw what they perceived as greener grass on the other side of the fence, and it didn't matter if they had two yoke around their necks, they were determined to go and eat what they thought was greener grass on the other side of the fence.

I have seen commercials on television that are advertising jewelry sales and it shows a young man and a young woman eating at a nice restaurant with soft lighting sitting across from each other; and then suddenly the man pulls out of his pocket a little box and opens it and there in that box is a beautiful shiny diamond ring and he looks at his girlfriend and asks "will you marry me." At that moment the cameras zero in on the girlfriends eyes which are now riveted on the beautiful shiny diamond ring and she breaks out into a beautiful and radiant smile and responds "yes". That commercial somehow gives the impression that she is saying yes to the ring not to the young man.

Now please don't miss understand me. I'm not putting down wedding rings or jewelry; just make sure you understand that a wedding ring will not keep you true to your wedding vows.

We have become a nation so dependent upon medications and drugs that we need a drug to get us going in the morning; we need a drug to keep us going through the day; and we need a drug to get to sleep on, and this vicious cycle continues until our mind tells our bodies, "I'm checking out; I can't take this any longer," and many times, we collapse under the stress.

Chapter Ten: Cancer

Almost everyone reading this book has a family member or close friend or at least knows someone who has had cancer or has cancer now.

Cancer is no respecter of persons. The very wealthy and the poor all succumb to cancer. I can remember when my wife and I were living in Gentry, Arkansas, about forty-five minutes from where Sam Walton lived, the founder of Wal-Mart. News got out that Sam had cancer. It was devastating to his family, as it is to all families who have to face dealing with a loved one or close friend who is going through cancer treatment.

Why did Sam come down with cancer? I'm sure his wife, kids, friends, and many business associates asked the same question. I certainly don't know; but there are three areas from which I believe cancer arises or any combination of the three:

- Heredity
- Environment
- Lifestyle

Remember earlier in the this book I shared with you a quote from Doctor Murdock of Loma Linda University in California. I want to quote it here again: "Faulty genetics loads the gun; lifestyle pulls the trigger."

Complex diseases are the result of genetic and environmental events; but even with complex diseases, making simple lifestyle changes can alleviate symptoms of the diseases and reduce the amount or dosage of medication you may be taking, or you may have to take for the remainder of your life.

Can we change our genetics? Not really, but we may be able to change our environment and we can definitely change our lifestyle.

I was adopted when I was three years old and although later in life as an adult I visited my biological mother;, I never had the opportunity to meet my biological father. Maybe had I been able to spend some time with him, I may have understood why I am hell bent on certain things and then to know what diseases or medical issues I may be facing in the future.

Now, I could say, "Well, I don't know what disease I might have lying dormant in my cells," and begin to worry until the stress from the worry actually brings on disease. In my situation, lifestyle will make the biggest difference and have the greatest impact for me, and that is true for you and for everyone. Isn't that good news.

When you make all the lifestyle changes you can, then you can safely relax knowing you have done everything you can to promote good health. And if you institute these changes early enough in your life and your children follow your lead, in a couple of generations your family will have some strong genetics. This is where I say you have a responsibility to change your DNA. This is how you do it—one lifestyle change at a time, one generation at a time.

The question becomes how much you are willing to sacrifice in your life to ensure your posterity has strong genetics; and honestly, you'll find it isn't a sacrifice at all. You certainly live longer and therefore have many more healthy years of life to share with your children, grandchildren, and maybe even great grandchildren.

I would be remiss if I didn't include this: Making changes in your lifestyle will not only make your children stronger physically, it will also make them stronger mentally and morally.

This week, I was browsing the internet and came upon a report that Joni Eareckson has breast cancer. After diving into shallow water as a young girl, Tada was rendered paralyzed (as a *quadriplegic*; unable to use her hands or legs).After two years of rehabilitation and in a wheelchair, Tada began working to help others in similar situations.

That was in 1967 when she was only eighteen years of age. She is now sixty. She has authored over thirty-five books. She has a radio talk show. She is a singer and painter and a movie has been made of her life. Now I don't know her, but I do know that no matter what hereditary baggage she arrived with when she was born certainly didn't stop Joni from accomplishing incredible things.

Thank you so much, Joni, for the encouragement you give to so many people who think they are in an inescapable situation of circumstances that they must resign themselves to.

"No, no, no," I want to cry out to every person reading this book that no matter what the hereditary genes you were given when you came into this world, there is always hope. You just have to know where to find it. That is the "naked truth."

Environment, on the other hand, is something that we may not be able to do anything about. For instance, as children, where our parents decide to live and the lifestyle they decide to follow or they adopt we probably don't have a great say in. One of the things that really bothers me is to see a parent, mom or dad, with a baby or child riding in the car and the parent is smoking and the windows are rolled up. No, I don't believe it's okay to smoke with a child in the car or anyone in the car just because the windows are down. Talk about child abuse. It is almost a terrorist mentality on the part of the parent. The terrorist isn't just killing himself or herself, he or she is also destroying innocent people.

A couple bumper stickers I saw recently caught my attention about our beautiful American flag. "These colors don't run." "If you want to burn the American flag, wrap yourself in it first." America, we have to get back to what this country was founded upon. We have to take back our health from the drug cartels that are legally wrecking the lives of millions of Americans everyday by the poisons they are dispensing; and shame on you, FDA, for allowing these drugs to be manufactured and prescribed. The FDA, the pharmaceutical companies, the National Cancer Institute and, yes, our government are all more concerned about making money and about having control over people's lives than they are about the health and welfare of the people.

Years ago in the late eighties, I was conducting a "breath free" seminar formerly known as a stop smoking seminar for those who desired to kick the tobacco habit and addiction. The first night I always ask the participants to pick a date when they would actually stop smoking. They were then encouraged to bring all their remaining cigarettes and smoking or drug paraphernalia like their cigarette lighters and ashtrays to the seminar and dispose of them there as a public witness that they were really quitting. Everyone would give a round of applause when this happened and that greatly encouraged the person or persons who had made the decision to quit.

In particular, I remember one salesman who attended that seminar. He had been a smoker for over forty years. His wife was an RN at the hospital I administered anesthesia in and she worked in the recovery room taking care of the patients coming out of surgery. After surgery, I would take my patient to the recovery room and give a report to her and so I got to know about her and her family. She had heard I was holding a "breath free" seminar and asked her husband to attend and so he came to my seminar. She was now suffering from the second hand smoke she had been breathing for years and by no choice of her own and of course the third hand smoke that was in all the furnishings, drapery, carpet, and automobile.

The first couple of nights of the "breath free" seminar most everyone had made a decision to stop smoking by setting a date to bring their cigarettes, ashtrays, and cigarette lighters and throw them away in front of everyone. I knew from past seminars a lot of these people would also go back to their smoking within a very short time. Finally, on about the fourth night, the salesman came up to the front and informed me he was quitting smoking that night. He threw all his tobacco paraphernalia away at that moment. We tried to keep in contact with those who had attended the seminars and at the end of one year they would receive a diploma if they were still a nonsmoker. Well, before that year was over, I took a new position and my family and I relocated to another state. But about at a year later, we came back and closed on our house and I visited the salesman and his wife. The wife was elated and told me that her husband was still a nonsmoker.

Sometimes in changing your environment, you may have to take some drastic measures. In 2008, I was practicing anesthesia at St. Joe Hospital in Denver, Colorado. It was a busy practice on the O.B. floor. There was a scrub tech who I worked with in surgery when we would do c-sections. She was in her early twenties, single, and lived with her parents. Both her parents smoked and drank and she was now a smoker by her own choice; but one day when she came to work, she informed me she had stopped smoking. I told her congratulations and I shared with her some points on how to continue to be a nonsmoker.

St. Joe Hospital has a strict policy on smoking. No one is permitted to smoke in the hospital or even on the premises outside. You had to be on the opposite side of the sidewalk to smoke, you know, on the grassy part between the sidewalk and the street curb. So before this young girl decided to quit the nicotine addiction, I would see her outside sitting on the street curb smoking; so it was refreshing now not to see her there when I would take a walk around the hospital. But after a couple of months I was walking outside around the hospital and there she was smoking. I didn't want to embarrass her but our eyes met and I could tell she didn't want me to see her smoking. It was amazing to see how happy she had looked over those two months when she was not smoking, how much brighter her complexion was, how much more beautiful her smile had become and now how unhappy and sad she seemed that she was smoking again. I knew what it was. She felt she was a failure because she was smoking again.

A couple of days later, we met at the coffee and water area and she opened up and told me it was just too much to quit while living with her parents who both smoke and drink. I first encouraged her that she hadn't failed; actually, I explained to her that you can't fail unless you quit and that is why quitting is so depressing because you feel you have failed; but I reassured her that she hadn't failed. Then I told her that if she truly wanted to kick the habit, she needed a change in her environment and if that meant moving out of her parent's home—then she must do it. Hereditary was not her biggest problem. It was her environment.

If you go to your local nursery and buy a tiny oak tree that they have in one of those clay or plastic pots and take it home and sit it outside on your patio to enjoy, how big will that oak tree grow? It will only reach to the height its environment allows it to—which might be about four feet. But if you remove that little oak tree from that pot and plant it outside where it has unlimited room and receives plenty of sunlight and rain, it will reach heights as great as forty feet and more. What makes the difference? The environment is the deciding factor, not the parent tree from which it came from.

We cheat ourselves when we say, "Well, my mother or my daddy had high "blood pressure or diabetes so I'll have the same diseases as they have," but that just isn't true if you make some simple lifestyle changes for yourself. You have a responsibility to make changes for those who may follow after you.

I have friends and others that I've met through my friends and many patients who say when they discover something they're eating, drinking, or doing in their life is causing them harm, "I'm going to die anyway so why worry about it." But what is interesting is you never hear one person mouth those words when they find themselves in ICU gasping for air, or holding their chest experiencing excruciating chest pain.

I've heard many men and some women who are imbibed say those words; but take away the alcohol and let their alcoholic saturated brain dry out and their tune will often change. Nobody wants to die, especially if one knows it's a choice that has brought him or her to where he or she is now.

Drinking alcohol beclouds the mind, especially the reasoning in the frontal lobe of the brain. I read somewhere how even one drink of alcohol can stay in the frontal lobe of the brain for up to two weeks.

Parents, don't buy into the idea that it's okay for your kids to drink alcohol at home and call that responsible drinking—there is no such thing as responsible drinking of any alcoholic beverages. That's an oxymoron. It's one thing for your children to learn to drink alcohol from other people, as sad as that is, but it's altogether different at the end of the day if your son or daughter becomes another statistic who was killed in an auto accident where alcohol was involved. It's hard to sleep at night with that on your mind.

I want to tell everyone, especially young people, to live a life without regrets as far as is within your power to do so.

Imagine when you were just a teenager or if you are that age now and in front of you there were, or are, five doors facing you. On the front of the first door is written alcohol; the second door, drugs; the third door, tobacco; the fourth door, pornography; and the fifth door, premarital sex.

Now, you may not know at the time whether your mom or dad, or an uncle or aunt, or a grandpa or grandma, is or was addicted to what's behind one of these doors. If you make a decision and exercise your will or power of choice and do not open one of these doors, you will never experience regret—at least in these areas; but if you do open one or, God forbid, all of these doors, you also don't know whether you will become an addict to the vice that's behind one of these doors.

I have known too many couples who have ended up in a divorce because of the blame game and jealousy. Premarital sex is at the core of this issue. When one or both parties in a marriage have had sex with someone else than the one they're married to now, feelings of jealousy and resentment take over where love for just one person should reign, and this becomes one of the greatest regrets of many young married couples.

When it's all said and done, after a divorce has taken place, at the end of the day, stress is the culprit that has finally triumphed.

I have read and heard on the news of numerous accounts of a drunk driver who crossed the yellow line and ran head on into an oncoming car. Many times, whole families are wiped out in a drunk driving crash. If people are killed in an automobile accident where alcohol is involved, the drunk driver is usually charged with manslaughter; the courts do not excuse the drunk driver because his brain was confused. The drunk driver, before he took a drink that finally ended in a fatal car accident, made a conscious choice to drink. Nobody forced him. Alcoholism is no disease, but it will cause disease. If alcoholism were truly a disease, the courts would be unjust for charging someone with manslaughter after killing a family because he was intoxicated. So alcoholism is not a disease; it's a choice.

Some look with horror upon men who have been overcome with liquor, and are seen reeling and staggering in the street, while at the same time they are gratifying their appetite for things differing in their nature from spirituous liquor but which injure the health, affect the brain, and destroy their high sense of spiritual things.

The liquor-drinker has an appetite for strong drink that he gratifies by drinking, usually more than he or she should, while another has no appetite for intoxicating drinks to restrain, but he desires some other hurtful indulgence, and does not practice self-denial any more than the drunkard.

Most people associate alcohol abuse with two diseases. The first is alcoholism, which is a syndrome of dependency that some believe is inherited. I don't believe alcoholism is a disease but I do believe you inherit the gene that gives you the propensity or the desire or the drive to drink. The other is cirrhosis, a disease that can be brought on by excessive alcohol consumption; but there are a number of other diseases and conditions that can develop, including pancreatitis, hypertension, osteoporosis and Wernicke-Korsakoff syndrome, just to mention a few:

1. Cirrhosis
    - Cirrhosis is essentially a scarring of the liver. Healthy tissue of the liver is replaced with fibrosis, or scar tissue. As this scar tissue builds up, it prevents the liver from functioning properly, which can lead to bile build up in the blood. Clotting may lessen and blood pressure may rise. Some of the most common symptoms of cirrhosis include lack of appetite, accompanied by weight loss, nausea, fatigue, jaundice, cognitive impairment (confusion and lack of concentration), tremors, internal bleeding, and coma.

2. Pancreatitis
    - Another common disease associated with alcohol abuse is pancreatitis, characterized by an inflammation of the pancreas and, much like cirrhosis, ultimate scarring of the organ. This scarring affects the production of insulin and the way in which sugar is released into the bloodstream. It often presents itself with severe abdominal pain that is typically accompanied by vomiting or nausea, the sweats, and a fever.

3. Hypertension
    - While more of a condition than a disease, hypertension, or high blood pressure, is another result of alcohol abuse. This condition is distinguished by essentially too much blood being forced through the arteries, which can damage the walls of these arteries and lead to a stroke, heart disease, heart attack, angina, pulmonary edema, and an aneurysm. Though high blood pressure is often seen as a hereditary condition, it can present itself in someone without a family history and even worsen hypertension in someone predisposed to it through genetics.

4. Osteoporosis
    - One of the most surprising diseases caused by alcohol abuse is osteoporosis, which involves the thinning of the bones or loss of bone mass. This depletion makes bones more brittle. While osteoporosis is most common in women, it can affect men, and excessive use of alcohol can diminish the vitamins and minerals needed for *healthy* bones, as well as exacerbate the effects of someone developing osteoporosis.

5. Wernicke-Korsakoff Syndrome
    - This brain disorder is a serious condition that can be caused by alcohol abuse. Essentially, this condition is a combination of two disorders that develop from a *vitamin* deficiency and an actual change in the brain. Typically, people who suffer from Wernicke-Korsakoff

> syndrome will experience blurred vision, memory loss, confusion, and problems with mobility, usually isolated to the legs. Sadly, a portion of this syndrome (that which involves the brain) can be permanent

Eliminating alcohol entirely from your life is a wise choice for your body, mind, and pocketbook. Remember, alcohol can remain in your system for two weeks. It continues to affect the frontal lobe of the brain, which is the reasoning center. So if your brain is soaked with alcohol, you won't always make good sound decisions. Your reflexes are not as quick. Alcohol can fool you into making you think you are handling things really well, because now that you have a couple drinks a day, you feel laid back and nothing bothers you. Others may admire you for your "cool hand luck" style of handling life; but make no mistake, you are never totally in control when you drink alcohol.

Many people who imbibe a couple of drinks a day are really alcoholics, but they just don't know it. When I was living and working in Colorado in about 2003, I got to know one of the PA's or physician assistants. He was a nice guy, had children, and a nice wife. They were probably in their late twenties to early thirties. He shared with me that he and his wife drank almost every night, not much he said, just maybe a couple of beers a night. I told him, "You're an alcoholic already and you don't know it."

He said, "No, I don't think so, I don't have to drink, I can quit anytime if I want to."

I challenged him to quit at least for a month. I said if you don't experience any withdrawal symptoms, then you're not yet an alcoholic. He never would take me up on the challenge. It gave him food for thought, though, because he later told me he and his wife had decided to cut back on their drinking.

Because alcohol affects the frontal lobe or the reasoning portion of the brain, you can be fooled into thinking that you are just a social drinker and you are quite in control and can stop drinking any time you want to.

I know many people who are very successful in life who have a drink or two when they want and seem to be enjoying life. Their marriage is successful, their children are doing well, they have money in the bank, and everything appears okay.... I can't and I won't argue that; but I'm really concerned about the person who has never taken a drink and doesn't know when he takes his or her first drink as to whether he or she will become the next alcoholic.

Unlike smoking, alcohol isn't so nauseating that you have to breathe the smoke from someone's cigarette; that is, unless you happen to bump into the town drunk or that social drinker that comes across the centerline and slams head on into your car and escapes without an injury but all your family are killed in your car. Then the town drunk, "Otis," as portrayed on the *Andy Griffith* show as a nice drunk who didn't even have a car and who never worked, isn't such a nice guy anymore. Hollywood can really glamorize the alcoholic, but that doesn't change the Naked Truth that alcohol is a killer, a family wrecker, a financial breaker, and many times a homeless maker.

Many people would say, "Don't you believe in moderation?" Absolutely! I believe in moderation in everything that is good; but for pornography, alcohol, tobacco, drugs, premarital sex, moderation does not apply. To truly be safe, abstinence is the key.

If you are so fortunate to have a beautiful daughter and she is attending high school or college, do you think moderation in premarital sex would be in order for your little girl? After all, some argue, we should do everything in moderation.

Chapter Eleven: AIDS

What is HIV? What is AIDS?

HIV (human immunodeficiency virus) is a virus that attacks the immune system, the body's natural defense system. Without a strong immune system, the body has trouble fighting off disease. Both the virus and the infection it causes are called HIV.

White blood cells are an important part of the immune system. HIV invades and destroys certain white blood cells, CD4+ cells. If too many CD4+ cells are destroyed, the body can no longer defend itself against infection.

The last stage of HIV infection is *AIDS* (acquired immunodeficiency syndrome). People with AIDS have a low number of CD4+ cells and get infections or cancers that rarely occur in healthy people. These can be deadly.

But having HIV does not mean you have AIDS. Even without treatment, it takes a long time for HIV to progress to AIDS—usually ten to twelve years. If HIV is diagnosed before it becomes AIDS, medicines can slow or stop the damage to the immune system. With treatment, many people with HIV are able to live long and active lives.

What Causes HIV?

HIV infection is caused by the human immunodeficiency virus. You can get HIV from contact with infected blood, *semen*, or vaginal fluids.

- Most people get the virus by having unprotected sex with someone who has HIV.
- Another common way of getting the virus is by sharing drug needles with someone who is infected with HIV.
- The virus can also be passed from a mother to her baby during pregnancy, birth, or breast-feeding.

HIV doesn't survive well outside the body, so it cannot be spread by casual contact such as kissing or sharing drinking glasses with an infected person.

What Are the Symptoms?

HIV may not cause symptoms early on. People who do have symptoms may mistake them for the flu or mono. Common early symptoms include:

- Fever
- Sore throat
- Headache
- Muscle aches and joint pain
- Swollen glands (swollen lymph node)
- Skin rash

Symptoms may appear from a few days to several weeks after a person is first infected. The early symptoms usually go away within two or three weeks.

After the early symptoms go away, an infected person may not have symptoms again for many years. Without treatment, the virus continues to grow in the body and attack the immune system. After a certain point, symptoms reappear and then remain. These symptoms usually include:

- Swollen lymph nodes
- Extreme tiredness
- Weight loss
- Fever
- Night sweats

A doctor may suspect HIV if these symptoms last and no other cause can be found.

Treatment usually keeps the virus under control and helps the immune system stay healthy.

Acquired Immunodeficiency Syndrome (AIDS) is the final stage of HIV infection. Lifestyle changes could eliminate HIV infection altogether. If we eliminate HIV infection, AIDS will cease to exist. Lifestyle is everything when it comes to overcoming AIDS for those who have received AIDS through lifestyle choices they have made.

Are you sick and tired of being sick and tired of your lifestyle? Do you want to get up in the morning feeling ready to meet the day without taking some drug or drinking something to get you started? Do you want to go through the day with all the energy you need without taking a stimulant? And, finally, do you want to go to bed and sleep through the night without taking a sleeping aid?

Well, reader, you can live a full and happy life by just making some simple lifestyle changes; and you won't be sick and tired of being sick and tired. You will realize that when you do get sick, it's usually your mind telling your body you need rest or a change in pace.

Neal Nedley, M.D., in his book *Proof Positive* writes about the following study:

Longevity Studies Related to Lifestyle

Just what are these lifestyle factors that will help us to live a longer life? Drs. Nedra Belloc and Lester Breslow were among the first researchers to present a convincing answer. In their classic study of nearly 7000 individuals living in Alameda County, California, they found that there were seven lifestyle factors that influenced how long people lived.

- ➢ 1. Sleep seven to eight hours
- ➢ 2. No eating between meals
- ➢ 3. Eat breakfast regularly
- ➢ 4. Maintain proper weight
- ➢ 5. Regular exercise
- ➢ 6. Moderate or no use of alcohol
- ➢ 7. No smoking

The number of habits that individuals followed made a tremendous impact on their longevity. After nine years, the number of healthful lifestyle practices a person followed was directly related to the likelihood of dying.

Relation of Longevity To Health Habits

Age-adjusted death rate

Men		Women	
No. of health habits practiced	Percent dead in 9 years	No. of health habits practiced	Percent dead in 9 years
7	5.5	7	5.3
6	11.0	6	7.7
5	13.4	5	8.2
4	14.1	4	10.8
0-3	20.0	0-3	12.3

Notice that only about 5 percent of men and women who followed all seven health habits died in the nine-year period, compared to 12.3 to 20 percent who followed three habits or less.

Another way of looking at the impact of lifestyle on longevity is by considering something referred to as "health age." As an example, a fifty-year-old who embraces enough healthful lifestyle factors may have the same health or physiologic age as the average thirty-five-year-old person. We could say that this individual has a "health age" of thirty-five. On the other hand, another fifty-year-old who had no regard for a healthful lifestyle may have a much older health age, perhaps as high as seventy-two. In other words, a person's health age can be lower or higher than the actual chronological age, depending on the number of lifestyle factors adopted."

Health age tables have been created from the Alameda County statistics. They cover the chronological age range from twenty years to seventy, and are based on the same seven health habits listed above. I would encourage you to purchase a copy of Proof Positive by Neil Nedley, M.D. Dr. Nedley covers in detail what I am writing about concerning your health age and many other issues dealing with healthful living.

You can use this figure as a guide to get a feel for your own health age. For example, assume that you are an average forty-year-old Alameda county resident. If you are following only two of the seven Belloc and Breslow's health habits, your health age is forty plus 19.4, or about fifty-nine, indicating a dramatic shortening of your life expectancy. You would have the same life expectancy as the average individual nineteen years older. If you continue the same lifestyle for ten more years, when you are fifty, your health age will be fifty plus twenty-two, or seventy-two. At age forty, you had a nineteen-year health handicap, but at age fifty, the handicap will even be worse by three years. In ten years, you will age thirteen years.

On the other hand, if you, at forty, are consistently following all seven of Belloc and Breslow's health habits, your health age is only twenty-seven (minus 12.9). Furthermore, at age fifty, your health age will be only thirty-five. In ten years, you will only age eight years! The concept of health age illustrates how much our lifestyle can either hasten or slow the aging process.

Early in this book, I mentioned a group of people who are known as Seventh-Day-Adventists and I stated I would say more about them later concerning their health practices.

The Seventh-Day-Adventists are a Christian group of people who have been practicing healthful living for over a hundred and fifty years. Their lifestyle is much more than just eating the right foods. They encourage a plant-based diet, but if you do eat meat, they maintain you should only eat clean meat. What is clean meat? In the Bible clean and unclean meats are succinctly written down. One of the main unclean meats mentioned in the Bible is pork. The Bible also gives many general health principles that if adopted would add years to your life.

The clean and unclean meats can be found in the Old Testament of the Bible in the book of Leviticus chapter eleven, beginning in verse one.

Seventh Day Adventists have always taught to anybody who has a desire to make changes in his or her lifestyle the way of life they have been living for over a hundred and fifty years. One of the first arguments by many on the subject of clean and unclean meats is that it no longer applies because in the New Testament of the Bible in the book of Acts chapter ten, it records an event that happened to Peter, a disciple and apostle of Jesus Christ.

According to Holy Scripture in the book of Acts chapter ten beginning with verse one, it reads, "On the next day, as they went on their journey and came near the city, Peter went up on the housetop to pray about noontime." This was not unusual in Bible times where Peter lived. Many of the houses were of adobe structures with flat roofs, a stairway where you could climb and, a parapet protecting you there while you read, prayed, or meditated—a place of quiet repose.

> And Peter became very hungry, and would have eaten: but while they were making lunch, he had a vision.
>
> He saw heaven opened, and a certain vessel descending to him, which had a great sheet knit at the four corners, and it was let down to earth.
>
> All kinds of four footed beasts of the earth, and wild beasts, and creeping things, and fowls of the air were in this sheet.
>
> And there came a voice to him, rise, Peter, kill, and eat. But Peter said, 'Not so, Lord; for I have never eaten anything that is common or unclean.'
>
> And the voice spoke unto him again the second time: "What God hath cleansed, don't call it unclean or common.
>
> This was done three times, and then the vessel was taken back into heaven. Now, while Peter doubted in what he had seen what it all meant, some men who were sent by a well-known gentile Cornelius stood before the house in which Peter was residing.
>
> Evidently, this Cornelius had also had a vision and was instructed to find Peter and ask him to come to his house and explain the gospel to him and his

> household. Well, Peter goes to Cornelius's house and says to him, "...You know how that it is an unlawful thing for a man that is a Jew to keep company, or come unto one of another nation; but God has shown me that I should not call any man unfit, uncommon or unclean."

Because of this text, many Christians defend their right to eat unclean meats like pork; but it has nothing to do with food. It has everything to do with treating everyone equally.

What is interesting is *The China Study* also recommends returning to a plant-based diet.

For a hundred and fifty years, Seventh Day Adventists have been sharing with millions of people the benefits of returning to a plant-based diet. They live longer and healthier lives. It is one thing to live until the age of sixty, seventy, or eighty dragging an oxygen tank around with you, but it is entirely different to still be able to climb mountains in your eighties and not to be toting around an oxygen tank.

Seventh Day Adventists are avid students of the Bible and follow the biblical teachings on healthful living.

In the book of Genesis chapter two, you find that the original diet God provided for mankind was plant based; and like The China Study and many other sources available, they encourage returning to a plant-based diet. It is a far superior diet, physically and mentally and provides protection from many diseases common to man today.

In the Bible in the book of Daniel of the Old Testament if you turn to the first chapter, you'll find a story that took place in the year 605 B.C....

Nebuchadnezzar, king of Babylon, besieged the city of Jerusalem and finally captured it and took most of the Jews back to Babylon. Babylon was the strongest nation at that time and King Nebuchadnezzar wanted to rule the world. So to advance his kingdom, he took some of the brightest youth who had been captured from Jerusalem and placed them in his university to educate them in the ways of the Chaldeans.

There was a young man, Daniel, who had three friends he associated with. This three were probably in their late teens, part of this group who were taken captive and were to be educated in the king's university. Their education lasted for three years and upon graduation , the king himself would give an oral examination.

Daniel and his three friends were raised not to eat any unclean meat and not to drink any alcoholic beverages. They were taught not to take anything into their bodies that was injurious to their health. Again, the Seventh Day Adventists go to the Bible for their guide in healthful living. In the New Testament, 1 Corinthians, and in chapter six and verse nineteen, it reads,

> What? Don't you know that your body is the temple of the Holy Ghost which is in you, which you have from God and you don't own your body.
>
> But you were bought with a great price; therefore glorify God in your body, and in your spirit, which are God's.

So healthful living for Seventh Day Adventists is a way of life for them; it's as natural as getting up in the morning.

In the book of Daniel chapter one, it says:

> But Daniel purposed in his heart that he would not defile himself with the portion of the king's meat, nor with the wine which he drank: therefore, he requested of the prince of the eunuchs that he might not defile himself.
>
> Now God had brought Daniel into favor and tender love with the prince of the eunuchs.
>
> And the prince of the eunuchs said unto Daniel, I fear my Lord the king, who hath appointed your food and your drink: for why should he see your faces worse liking than the children which are of your age? Then shall you make me endanger my head to the king.
>
> Then said Daniel to Melzar, whom the prince of the eunuchs had set over Daniel, and his three friends, Hananiah, Mishael, and Azariah.

> Test your servants, I beseech you, ten days; and let them give us beans to eat, and water to drink.
>
> Then let our countenances be looked upon before you, and the countenance of the children that eat of the portion of the king's food: and as you see, deal with your servants.
>
> So he consented to them in this matter, and tested them ten days.
>
> And at the end of ten days, their countenances appeared fairer and better looking than all the children who ate of the portion of the king's meat.
>
> Thus Melzar took away the portion of their meat, and the wine that they should drink; and gave them beans.
>
> As for these four children, God gave them knowledge and skill in all learning and wisdom: and Daniel had understanding in all visions and dreams.
>
> Now, at the end of the days (when their three years at the Babylonian university was finished) the king had said he should bring them in, then the prince of the eunuchs brought them in before Nebuchadnezzar.
>
> Daniel, Hananiah, Mishnael, and Azariah: therefore they served before the king.
>
> And in all matters of wisdom and understanding, that the king inquired of them, he found them ten times better than all the magicians and astrologers that were in all his realm.

It's quite a story and Seventh Day Adventists believe anyone can enjoy better physical and mental health like Daniel and his three friends did by returning to a plant based diet.

By the way, Daniel lived to be in his eighties and was very successful throughout his entire life.

A plant-based diet strengthens your immune system against many diseases, including cancer. Your mind is clearer. You wake up happier. You just look and feel better.

One of the most prolific writers of the 1800's was a woman by the name of Ellen White. She was impressed with the temperance society of her day and what they were trying to accomplish. She wrote books on health and advocated getting back to a plant-based diet. She wrote of the unhealthful practices of taking drugs for healing and of the dangers of caffeine, tobacco, and alcohol, and of many other harmful products popular then and are today.

Seventh Day Adventists call what Ellen White wrote on health "the health message."

Over a hundred years ago, she wrote this about tea and coffee:

> Tea acts as a stimulant, and to a certain extent, produces intoxication. The action of coffee and many other popular drinks is similar. The first effect is exhilarating. The nerves of the stomach are excited; these convey irritation to the brain, and this, in turn, is aroused to impart increased action to the heart and short-lived energy to the entire system. Fatigue is forgotten; the strength seems to be increased. The intellect is aroused, the imagination becomes more vivid.
>
> Because of these results, many suppose that their tea or coffee is doing them great good. But this is a mistake. Tea and coffee do not nourish the system. Their effect is produced before there has been time for digestion and assimilation, and what seems to be strength is only nervous excitement. When the influence of the stimulant is gone, the unnatural force abates, and the result is a corresponding degree of langor and debility."
>
> The continued use of these nerve irritants is followed by headache, wakefulness, palpitation of the heart, indigestion, trembling, and many other evils; for they wear away the life forces. Tired

> nerves need rest and quiet instead of stimulation and overwork.
>
> A practice that is laying the foundation of a vast amount of disease and even more serious evils is the free use of poisonous drugs. When attacked by disease, many will not take the trouble to search out the cause of their illness. Their chief anxiety is to rid themselves of pain and inconvenience.
>
> By the use of poisonous drugs, many bring upon themselves lifelong illness, and many lives are lost that might be saved by the use of natural methods of healing."

She wrote "popular nostrums called patent medicines"; I looked the up word "nostrums" in the dictionary and here is the definitions they gave:

1. a medicine sold with false or exaggerated claims and with no demonstrable value; quack medicine.
2. a scheme, *theory*, device, etc., especially one to remedy social or political ills; panacea.
3. a medicine made by the person who recommends it.
4. a patent medicine.

The above second definition caught my attention, "especially one to remedy social or political ills; panacea."

When President Obama became president, there was a "politically created scare" about the H1N1 becoming pandemic; but it was actually shown that more people died from the common flu that year than they did from the H1N1 virus.

But because of the hype, pharmaceutical companies were given billions of dollars for research for new vaccines and were given protection from any lawsuits that may arise if anyone died from receiving one of their vaccines.

If the government could have their way, they would place "drug medications" in the municipal water supply. I read somewhere that the government wants to put antihypertensive, and statin, and antidepressant in the city water supplies so high blood pressure, high cholesterol, and depression could be wiped out in America.

Is that the answer to the health problems in America? No, not at all.

Drug medication, as it is generally practiced, is a curse. We need to educate away from drugs.

Use drugs less and less, and depend more upon hygienic agencies; then nature will respond to God's physicians—pure air, pure water, proper exercise, a clear conscience. Then drugs would seldom need to be used.

We have become a drug dependent, drug crazed society. We take a drug to wake us up in the morning; we take drugs to keep us awake throughout the day, and, finally, we take a drug to put us to sleep at night.

So in looking at Seventh Day Adventists longevity of life, you find some common basic principles:

1. They eat mainly of a plant-based diet.
2 .They exercise regularly.
3. They do not eat any unclean meat.
4. They do not use tobacco, coffee, tea, or alcohol.
5. They rest one day a week on the seventh day or Saturday.
6. They are a very giving people in terms of helping others when disaster strikes.
7. They do not drink alcohol.

Unfortunately, not even all Seventh-Day-Adventist are putting into practice the ***Eight Natural Laws of Health.***

Some Seventh Day Adventists now drink alcohol and many drink coffee; but for those who are following fully the eight natural laws of health are truly reaping the benefits. As with everything else in life that we say or do, the old saying, "We reap what we sow" really applies when it comes to the lifestyle we choose to live.

I know many people who are actually practicing many of the eight laws of health and have never even heard of a Seventh Day Adventist. Anyone can reap the benefits that come from following the eight natural laws of health.

I have spent considerable space on the topic of alcohol and I want to recommend another book entitled *Wine in the Bible*, written by Dr. Samuele Bacchiocchi, who was professor of Church History and Theology at Andrews University, Berrien Springs, Michigan, when he wrote this book. In the next few paragraphs, I will be quoting some of his research he provides in this book.

Dr. Bacchiocchi passed away about four years ago for which I deeply regret. His son Daniele Bacchiocchi has given me permission to copy some material from his father's book, "Wine in the Bible"-A Biblical Study on the Use of Alcoholic Beverages. Thank you Daniele and family.

There is a "raging epidemic of alcohol use in American society in general and in my own Seventh Day Adventist church in particular. In American society, alcohol has become its number one public enemy, costing over $117 billion a year, disabling over 100,000 lives, 25 times as many as all illegal drugs combined. The real human cost of alcohol transcends these statistical figures of dollars, disabilities and death. No one can count the real cost of alcohol to our society in terms of retarded children, violence in the home, child and spouse abuse, divorce, rape, robberies, murders, sickness and death."

He continues:

> I soon became aware that Christian churches bear considerable responsibility for the alcohol epidemic. Through their beliefs, teachings, and preaching they are able to influence the moral values pastors preach from their pulpits on the subject of drinking determines to a large extent the stand Christians take toward alcoholic beverages. A majority of the 100 million drinkers in America are churchgoers who have been taught that the Bible sanctions a moderate use of alcoholic beverages. Moderate drinking has led over eighteen million Americans to become immoderate drinkers, for alcohol is a habit-forming narcotic, weakening one's capacity for self-control.

> Even Billy Graham, a teetotaler, said, 'I do not believe that the Bible teaches teetotalism...Jesus drank wine. Jesus turned water into wine at a wedding feast. That wasn't grape juice as some of them try to claim.
>
> The drinking of alcoholic beverages by over 100 million Americans is rightly regarded by social analysts as America's number one public enemy. The economic cost to the American society of the use of alcohol is estimated by the National Institute on Alcohol Abuse and Alcoholism at 117 billion a year. This staggering figure includes the cost of premature deaths, reduced production and special treatments.

He continues:

> Those who teach that moderate drinking is a Christian liberty sanctioned by Scripture fail to realize that moderation is the first step toward immoderation. First, because alcohol is a habit-forming narcotic and second, because even moderate drinking diminishes our capacity for judgment and self-control."
>
> Billy Graham caused a great uproar across the United States when he condoned President Carter's position to serve only wine at the White House, by saying: 'I do not believe that the Bible teaches teetotalism...Jesus drank wine. Jesus turned water into wine at a wedding feast. That wasn't grape juice as some of them try to claim." To calm the outcry from conservatives, Graham clarified his position, saying: "It is my judgment that because of the devastating problem that alcohol has become to America, it is better for Christians to be teetotalers except for medical purposes...The creeping paralysis of alcoholism is sapping our morals, wrecking our homes, and luring people away from the church.

Dr. Brocchciocchi continues:

> The reduction of alcoholism to the status of a disease to which some people are vulnerable began in the late 1930's and has become widely accepted. A reason for this is, as stated by San Francisco psychologist Paul Good, that 'if you call it a moral problem, you don't have a treatment industry.' He adds, 'A billion-dollar industry services alcoholism as a disease.' This flow of money into treatment programs-from employers, insurance companies and governments-could dry up quickly if the Supreme Court were to undermine alcoholism's status as disease."
>
> The adoption of the sickness model has largely eliminated the moral aspect of alcohol abuse, reducing it to a genetic and/or physiological disorder. This popular view is now being challenged by scholars such as Herbert Fingareette, an expert on addiction at the University of Southern California who is often consulted by the government in legal cases involving alcoholics. In his newly released book, Heavy Drinking: The Myth of Alcoholism as a Disease, Fingarette argues convincingly, on the basis of several recent medical studies which have been largely ignored, that heavy drinking is in most cases a behavioral rather than a medical problem."
>
> It is not surprising that alcoholism has been reduced to the status of sickness for which the individual is not responsible. This is simply another example of the fact that we are fast becoming a "no fault" society—a society where no one is willing to assume responsibility or blame for anything he does. We have no fault insurance and no fault divorces, so why not also have no fault alcoholism?

> Ralph Woerner perceptively observes: "Alcoholics are no longer to blame for what they have become. They have caught a disease, like chicken pox, measles or mumps. The poor fellow was thirsty. He went into a bar one day where they served him a disease causing drink, which destroyed his brain, wrecked his marriage, and brought untold anguish upon his family. But it was all so innocently done. No one is responsible for what happened."
>
> We would never allow a company to sell a beverage which causes measles, smallpox, or polio, but with alcohol it is different. When the consumer becomes addicted, he has contracted a disease. This 'schizophrenic' reasoning allows the manufacturer to sell his product without responsibility or blame. It allows the user to destroy himself without guilt or shame. He is a 'victim' like someone who has been hit by a tornado, an earthquake, or a flood. How can he be held responsible for what he has become? By labeling alcoholism a disease, we absolve the alcoholic of all responsibility and guilt.

Honestly, I don't believe many Seventh Day Adventists understand the gift they have been given through the health message given to them on a silver platter through the writings of Ellen White—probably the most prolific female writer of the nineteenth century.

Years ago, I used to listen to Paul Harvey regularly on the radio and every once in a while I would hear Paul say, "Ellen White once again has been proven correct by science." I'm paraphrasing, but the point was that what Ellen White wrote over a hundred years ago or more is now being proven by modern science. Here are a few examples:

Heavy suppers stymie weight loss

Ellen White's Words: "The last meal (supper) is generally the most hearty and is often taken just before retiring. This is reversing the natural order; a hearty meal should never be taken so late in the day."

Medical Science Speaks: Leaving off supper may be one of the best ways to deal with excess weight. One study documented weight loss in all of nearly 600 patients who ate their last meal no later than 3:00 P.M.

Warning against Sugar

Ellen White's Words: "From the light given me, sugar, when largely used, is more injurious than meat."

Medical Science Speaks: A number of different cancers have now been statistically linked to sugar consumption. The risk of more sugar is consumed: colon cancer, uterine cancer, prostate cancer, kidney cancer, and cancers of the nervous system.

Coffee is Hurtful:

Ellen White's Words: "Coffee is a hurtful indulgence. It temporarily excites the mind...but the aftereffect is exhaustion, prostration, paralysis of the mental, moral, and physical powers. Tea acts as a stimulant.... The action of coffee...is similar. Fatigue is forgotten, the strength seems to be increased...when the influence of the stimulant is gone, the unnatural force abates, and the result is a corresponding degree of languor and disability."

Medical Science Speaks: The internationally acclaimed Norwegian research project known as the Tromso heart study assessed 143,000 men and women and found a significant increase in depression in women who were heavy coffee users.

Caffeine addictiveness has only recently been proven at John Hopkins University. Researchers at John Hopkins published startling research that demonstrated that "caffeine has the cardinal features of a prototypic drug of abuse." Based on its drug effects, caffeine acts much like any classic addictive drug. The implication is that habitual caffeine users are as much drug addicts, in the chemical sense of the term, as cocaine addicts, heroin addicts, or nicotine addicts.

Ellen White also warned of its effect on the mind, which also has only recently been proven.

These above examples are just a few of the many you can find in Neil Nedley, M.D.'s book *Proof Positive*. This information is listed in the back of his book.

Ellen White wrote volumes on topics related to health, healing, and lifestyle. *Ministry of Healing, Counsels on Diet and Foods, Medical Ministry, and Counsels on Health* are four books that contain information and advice on a wide variety of diseases and conditions. These books and others have undergone many printings over the decades and are still available and in demand today.

Ask Seventh Day Adventist members; they will be able to tell you where you can buy any of her books. If you visit any of the many Adventist book stores across the United States, you will find her books.

George E. Vandeman, who also was a Seventh-Day-Adventist and who started and was the founder and first speaker of the *It Is Written Telecast*, a ministry that is still on television today, wrote a book entitled, *I Met a Miracle*, which was published in 1960.

George Vandeman was a preacher but he also encouraged people to make lifestyle changes to help them live a fuller, happier, and longer life.

SKIDDING ALONG! Getting by! Getting by with the aid of too many cups of coffee, too many cigarettes, too much wound-up nervous energy—and too little sleep, relaxation, fun, and frolic. Spending five dollars' worth of nervous energy on a five-cent problem. Tense, parchment-faced individuals who cannot decide whether to take a Benzedrine and go to a party or take a Seconal and go to bed!

An old legend tells of a Portuguese monastery that stood precariously atop a three-hundred-foot cliff. Visitors were strapped in a huge wicker basket, then pulled to the top with an old ragged rope. As one visitor stepped into the basket for the descent, he asked anxiously, "How often do you get a new rope?"

"Whenever the old one breaks," a monk replied.

Risky-dangerous-like skidding through life on a threadbare rope! Tired-ready to break!

In this hurry-scurry, pell-mell, atomic age of jets, speed, and spasm, we take too little time to live sanely. We careen down the wild highway of modern life until our health is gone. And then, with our time and with our money, we pay. Too late, we discover that when the rope breaks, it cannot be replaced. The Creator gave us only one.

It was back in 1925 that a young medical student at the German University of Prague, burning with enthusiasm for the art of healing, noticed what many physicians before him had noticed, that there are certain symptoms that are common to a great many diseases, and are therefore of little help in making diagnoses. For instance, the fact that a patient feels ill, has a slight fever, a loss of appetite, and a few scattered aches and pains, would hardly enable a physician to pinpoint the disease.

Young Hans Selye was too new in the medical profession to realize just how laughable his question might sound to his elders—if he should find the courage to ask it. But why, he wondered, had physicians since the dawn of medicine given their attention to understanding the specific symptoms of individual diseases and never troubled themselves to understand the condition of "just being sick?" What is it that makes a man sick—not sick with pneumonia, or sick with scarlet fever, or sick with measles, but just plain sick? Why could not the methods and instruments of research be applied to that problem?

That question in a pioneering young mind was the beginning of many years of research that have resulted in a most valuable contribution to modern science—the better understanding of the stress of life.

Stress, you see, is simply the wear and tear of life. It is what life does to you. Stress is not necessarily caused by some great problem that rolls suddenly upon the mind or body of man. It may be caused by crossing a street in traffic, by reading with poor light, by the ringing of the telephone, by an endless variety of routine everyday occurrences—even by sheer joy. It is not possible to avoid stress entirely. But it is possible, and very important, to adjust your reaction to it, to strengthen the body's defenses against it. For medical science now knows that many diseases are caused largely by errors in the body's response to stress, rather than by germs or poisons or any other outside agent.

One of Dr. Selye's most valuable, and most interesting, contributions has been to point out that every man begins life with a certain reserve of vital force, or adaptation energy. Once it is gone, it cannot be replaced. It is like a bank account that can be depleted by withdrawals but cannot be increased by deposits.

Many people use up this vitality, restore if from superficial supplies, and are tricked into thinking the loss has been made up by rest. On the contrary, every withdrawal of the deeper reserves of vital force leaves its scar. The man who thinks he can tax his body beyond normal limits and then restore it all by a few hours or a few days of rest is like the spendthrift who draws money out of his savings, puts it into his checking account, and reasons that no loss has been sustained.

The man deceives himself. For stress, somewhere, is wearing the defenses thin. The body is only as strong as its weakest part. And someday, like the rope at the Portuguese monastery, it will break.

Listen to this significant description of our day: "But understand this, that in the last days there will come times of stress. For men will be lovers of self, lovers of money, proud, arrogant, abusive, disobedient to their parents, ungrateful, unholy, inhuman, implacable, slanderers, profligates, fierce, haters of good treacherous, reckless, swollen with conceit, lovers of pleasure rather than lovers of God." 2 Timothy 3:1-4, R.S.V.

Stress in the last days. And every one of us has felt it. But tornadoes are not mentioned as the cause. Earthquakes are not blamed. The stress we feel is not the mysterious fallout of H-bombs. Stress comes from within.

But men and women do not want to look within. They are not content to lay their guilt and their grudges at the foot of an old-fashioned cross. A cross does not seem to fit into this pell-mell age. They look elsewhere to drown their restless boredom.

Tired—ready to break! But millions keep themselves awake, and keep themselves asleep, and try to solve their endlessly growing problems with a streamlined pill. They ignore nature's red light and careen blindly on.

Fatigue, you see, is nature's warning that vital energy is being exhausted. But men and women ignore the warning, put a penny in the fuse box by indulging in another cup of coffee, another cigarette, another pill—and carry on.

These are not idle words. The spine-chilling term drug addiction may be nearer to you and your family than you think.

Let us go back to World War II, when new drugs were discovered that gave their users abnormal strength and courage temporarily. The Allies, the Nazis, the Japanese, used them. They went into the kits of men sent on dangerous missions.

But tragedy occurred when with war's end these same drugs moved onto our highways to keep sleepy truck drivers awake. Then into the athletic lockers across America, and onto the playing fields to stimulate more spectacular performance. And finally, into the medicine cabinets of average American families.

These chemical crutches look innocent enough. The first one may make you feel like a miracle. But how does it make you feel to know that a surprising number of cars you meet on the highway are driven by mildly, or not so mildly, drugged persons—persons who, at any moment, may suddenly see things coming toward them that are not there? Death travels the concrete ribbons. And the intoxicant responsible may not be in a bottle at all, but in a streamlined pill!

Did you know that if a warehouse were stacked high with bags of ordinary coffee beans, there would not be an ounce of actual food value in the lot? Could it be that the millions of pounds of coffee consumed by Americans are only pennies in the fuse box, forcing tired bodies to carry on beyond their strength? Is there such a thing as coffee addiction? Many medical men are answering, "Yes."

Did it ever occur to you that the popularity of many cola drinks is not due to their flavor, or even to their tremendous advertising, but to the dose of caffeine they contain? And is afternoon tea only a pleasant custom? Try giving it up!

Tired—ready to break! Is it not time to ask, "What makes man tired?"

A book popular in our bookstores for some years bore the title How Never to Be Tired. It had a phenomenal sale because there are so many millions of tired people in the world.

Now the assertion that it is possible never to be tired obviously needs qualification. For there is a natural and normal tiredness that comes from physical labor. The wise man said that the sleep of a laboring man is sweet. And in John 4:6, we are told that Jesus was weary and found it necessary to rest.

A wholesome bodily weariness from hard work is quickly balanced. The energy lost during the day is built up with a good night's sleep. But there is a tiredness that is not so easily replaced—a tiredness that dips into the reserves of vital force.

What is it, then, that in this deeper sense makes you tired? A troubled mind—selfishness—worry—depression—fear—guilt—and the streamlined pill you take to try to correct them. All these make you tired. All these produce stress. All these break down the life forces and invite disease. All these can poison the springs of life.

You say, "All this is very startling. And I can see that it is true. But what can I do about it? How can I keep from passing on the tiredness of the mind to the body?

Thank God, there is an answer! And that answer is not, simply understanding the psychological aspects of the problem, however helpful that may be. Nothing will satisfy now except that which meets the simple, unadorned needs of the soul. You want a prescription for the strange, unsatisfied tiredness within.

Therefore, I offer you the invitation of the Saviour: "*Come unto me,...and I will give you rest.*"

Simple words. But they are the words of the Creator of the body and of the mind. These words, I sincerely believe, are a prescription for all the physical, mental, and spiritual ills of man. They may sound too simple to work. But they have never failed.

Is yours a tired body? The world offers its miracle drugs. But God says, "I will restore health unto thee, and I will heal thee."

Is yours a tired mind? Modern science knows how to jerk a tired mind out of a rut. But God says, "A new heart [a new mind] also will I give you."

Is yours a tired soul? There are voices that counsel you to silence the conscience, to forget your inhibitions, if you would be healed. But Jesus came to "save his people from their sins."

Rest! When you lay your guilt at the foot of the cross, you will find it. "If we confess our sins, He is faithful and just to forgive us our sins, and to cleanse us from all unrighteousness."

Rest! When you lay your selfishness at the foot of the cross, you will find it. "Whosoever will save his life shall lose it; but whosoever shall lose his life for my sake...shall save it."

Rest! When you lay your fear at the foot of the cross, you will find it. "Perfect love casteth out fear: because fear hath torment." Fear torments. Guilt poisons. Selfishness kills. But love heals!

Wow! What George Vandeman wrote back in 1960 is still applicable today.

Why do you suppose that is? I believe it is because basic tenets to good health, happiness, and longevity of life don't change.

In 2010, Haiti was hit with its worst earthquake ever, devastating the island around Port-a-Prince. A good friend of mine, Dr. Elias Hernandez, who I worked with in Colorado, called me at our new residence in Tennessee and said, "I'm putting a medical team together to go to Haiti and I need an anesthesia provider; would you join me; we're leaving in a week." Fortunately, I was able to get someone to work for me at the hospital.

Dr. Hernandez sent me an itemized list of things I needed to bring with me to Haiti. The main thing that caught my attention on the list was it said bring your own food. Water would be provided but not food.

My wife got together crackers, nuts, pecans, and almonds, and dried fruit-enough to last about a week. It was hot in Haiti at the time we were there. Dr. Hernandez and I slept in a mosquito netting under the stars and had a wonderful time giving medical aid to the Haitian people. We found the Haitian people to be a very happy and resilient people especially in light of what they had just experienced.

The reason I share this experience with you is to show you that I fared very well from the food I took to Haiti. If I had been accustomed to a stimulating diet of dairy foods, meat, coffee and soft drinks or power bars and power drinks, I don't think I would have done so well.

I remember watching the news on television during the Katrina hurricane in New Orleans and seeing the rescue of a rather large woman through a window and they had her on a piece of plywood and the rescuers were letting her down to safety.

When disasters like hurricanes, earthquakes, tornadoes, tsunami's, famines, pestilences, cholera, and dysentery strike America, are you ready physically and mentally to weather the storm?

More than one half of the world's population are in cities. Large food chains like Wal-Mart, Kroger's, and Publix's are re-stocked about every day and a half. That means most people living in the large cities are about nine meals or three days away from running out of food.

There is an agenda among world leaders today to build more cities—large cities, larger than we now have. Governments know if you want to control the people, you need to corral them into cities. Make the people totally dependent upon you, the government, for everything—food, water and all of your toiletries, then controlling the masses becomes much easier.

I firmly believe in the near future there will be a requirement for a visa if you want to travel from one state to another state within the *"Free"* United States; *the storm is coming—make no mistake; the question is, are you ready?*

The single greatest thing you can do for yourself and for your families is to get off drug-medications. Don't become dependent upon pharmaceutical companies or the drug cartels for your health and happiness, because good health, happiness, and longevity of life don't come from ingesting their poisons; good health, happiness, and longevity of life is the result of living within the natural laws of health that God instituted when He created man—it's as simple as that.

If you're growing old, please don't become a grumpy old person. Here are some ways to keep that from happening:

- Stretch when you get up in the morning and remain active.
- Develop a hobby.
- Do volunteer work.
- Read and memorize.
- Get rid of drug-medications. Ingesting a lot of medications can change your whole outlook on life.
- Be thankful and you will soar with the eagles

- Don't complain because I'm looking to you for some positive mentoring and encouraging words. Your experience and advice is valuable and very much needed in this generation.

A young man and his wife were sightseeing in Estes Park, Colorado walking past the storefronts when they encountered an elderly lady who asked, "How are you doing?"

The young man replied, "I can't complain."

"Good", responded the elderly lady. "Because I don't want to hear your complaints."

That young man told me that left a deep impression on his mind.

Are you growing (physically, mentally, spiritually) old or are you just growing old? There is a difference. That difference is: Are you active physically, mentally and spiritually.

I want to be running when I die, not rocking in a chair dosed up with drug-medications and having oxygen pumped into my lungs through a nasal cannula.

Many people ask me, "What fruits and vegetables should I eat?"

My response is always, "Eat what is indigenous to where you are living." If you eat a variety of fresh fruits and vegetables indigenous to your area and add to that legumes, nuts, and grains, and drink plenty of cool, fresh, spring water, you will get all the vitamins and protein you will ever need.

If you're one of those people who feel gassy and bloated after eating beans, then try this:

Soak your beans overnight, then throw away the water, followed by discarding the water with which you bring your beans to a boil; this will remove a lot of the soluble fiber. My wife also removes the white foam that is present when you bring your beans to a boil. She just takes a spoon and throws the white foam out.

The soluble fiber is what feeds the bacteria that may be causing the gas you are experiencing.

If beans still do not agree with you, don't eat them; there are plenty of foods that you can get your fiber from besides beans.

At the beginning of this book, I said I would speak more on the old adage, "Early to bed, early to rise, makes a man healthy, wealthy, and wise."

When you go to bed early and the more sleep you receive before midnight, more of those stress-reducing hormones, like serotonin and melatonin, are secreted.

I found these next three sentences on the internet written by Ed Clements on January of 2009:

> Serotonin has come under a lot of attention recently because research has shown that low levels of this neurotransmitter can lead to increased incidences of aggressive behavior and increased symptoms of anxiety and depression.
>
> Even more worryingly is that scientists have found that lower serotonin function and impulsive/aggressive traits are associated with suicidal acts, including completed suicide.
>
> Serotonin is a neurotransmitter that helps to regulate many functions in the body. Serotonin is the chemical that helps you to feel refreshed after a good night's sleep.

The main time during which your body receives serotonin is before midnight, so it's important you get to bed early. Wind down in the evening by taking a leisurely walk. When I'm home and if the kids are in bed asleep, my wife and I often take our little bishon for a walk through the neighborhood. We're not rushed because our dog stops about twenty times to lay down his scent, and so we just talk about the days' activities or about what lies ahead for tomorrow.

Don't wait to turn off the television in the evening just before you go to bed. I've read studies where they've shown that watching television just before going to bed can cause you to have a restless nights' sleep—contrary to popular opinion. They showed the same is true with computers.

Melatonin, another compound that is primarily secreted in your body before midnight, helps regulate sleep and wake cycles.

Several clinical studies indicate that supplementation with melatonin is an effective preventive treatment for migraines and cluster headaches.

So if you're waking up in the morning with a headache, with little energy, and just feeling lousy, you may be suffering from low levels of serotonin and melatonin. No, you don't need to run out and buy expensive serotonin and melatonin products; just eat more fresh fruits and vegetables and get more sleep before midnight. It's that simple. By making these simple lifestyle changes, you will begin waking up refreshed, with more energy and with fewer headaches.

The more rest you get before midnight, the more your brain is rested and you will not make so many stupid decisions and stupid choices that can lead to depression because you have so many regrets.

You have more energy to make it through the whole day without coffee or other drinks loaded with caffeine and without the caffeine, you will find yourself wanting to retire earlier.

And no matter what is happening in your environment around you, remember to wake up on the inside; don't let circumstances around you dictate how you will respond to what comes at you throughout the day. Don't let anything or anybody steal your joy. When you arise after a good nights' rest, determine that you are going to have a great day come what may, and you will.

Before my conclusion I have placed an article by Lisa Farino that I pulled off the internet from MSN's "Health and Fitness" which helps articulate some reasons for our happiness. Now while I strongly feel true happiness can only come from a power outside of our selves—-I believe that power is our Creator God.

The more of the eight laws of natural healing you incorporate into your lifestyle, the healthier you will be; this same rule applies when seeking happiness. If you are married, have a strong belief and attend religious services regularly, have good work ethics, are not a couch potato and do not think everyone owes you a free ticket to success, are involved in some form of giving from your money, talent and time, understand how to love people and use things, have an attitude of gratitude, take time to relax and laugh, then you will always be able to get up on the inside no matter what is happening on the outside. That is the Naked Truth.

1 of 10
< Previous | Next >

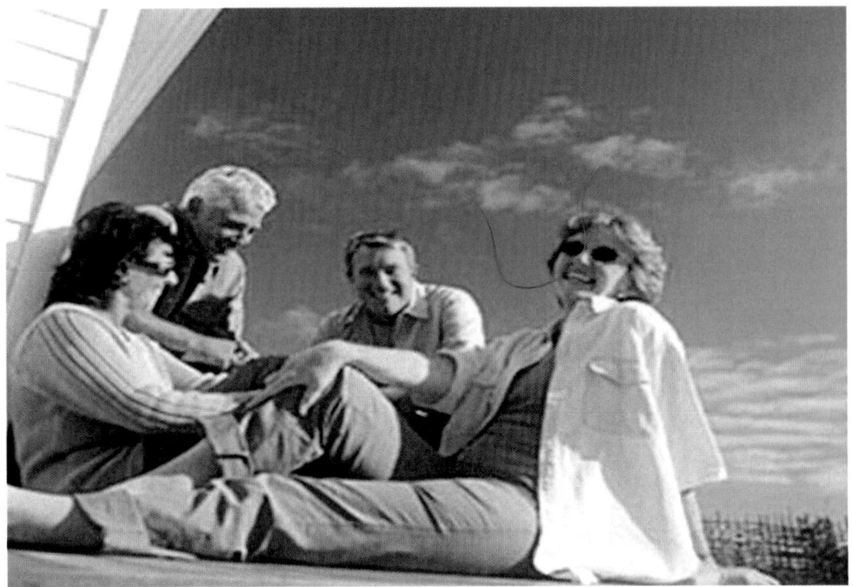

By Lisa Farino for MSN Health & Fitness

What Makes Us Happy?

In recent years, researchers have attempted to use a variety of statistics and surveys to answer a question that's occupied countless generations of philosophers: What makes us truly happy?

While some evidence suggests that happiness may be linked, in part, to relative wealth—how we're doing compared to those around us—overall, the old adage that money doesn't buy happiness seems to hold true.

"We are materially so much better off than we were fifty years ago, but we're not one iota happier," says Chris Peterson, a psychology professor at the University of Michigan.

That's no surprise to happiness expert, David Myers, who sees happiness as more closely correlated with people rather than things. "We humans have a deep need to belong—to connect with others in close, supportive, intimate, caring relationships," he says. "People who have such close relationships are more likely to report themselves 'very happy.'"

We've compiled a list of eight factors that influence rates of happiness and depression. Many of these factors vary from city to city and region to region. Here's your chance to see how your city compare.

How Happy Is Your City?

Content provided by: 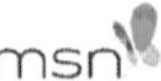

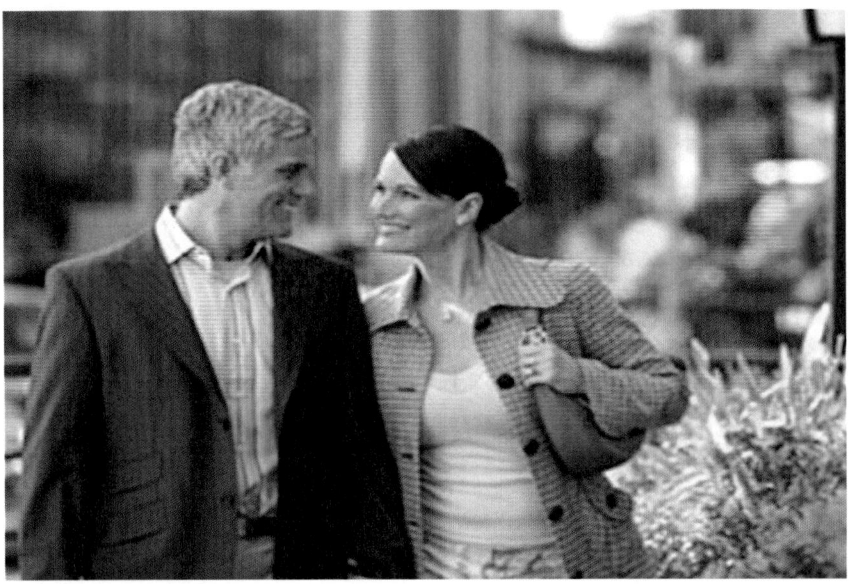

Happily Married

Is getting married one of the keys to a happy life? A 2006 report from the Pew Research Center suggests so—43 percent of married women and men reported being "very happy," while only 24 percent of unmarried men and women said the same.

Interestingly enough, the happy halo that shines over married couples isn't the result of having kids—those with children were just as likely to be happy as those without.

Rather, there seems to be something about marriage itself that boosts both men's and women's feelings of well-being in life.

"Recent research suggests that people become less depressed and less lonely after they get married," says Linda Waite, a sociology professor at the University of Chicago and author of *The Case for Marriage*.

After all, it's harder to be lonely when you've got a loved one to come home to every night.

According to Waite, men benefit even more than women from having a life-long companion. "Women will talk to everyone," says Waite, "But most men tend to rely on their wives as their main confidant."

In addition, women—typically the social planners in a relationship—ensure that the men stay connected to family and friends, another source of happiness.

And what about all that nagging that wives are so famous for? Turns out it pays off. Men who are married drink less, smoke less, eat better, get more sleep, and engage in less risky behavior than their unmarried peers. The end result: Married men are healthier, and since health is linked to happiness, they're happier, too.

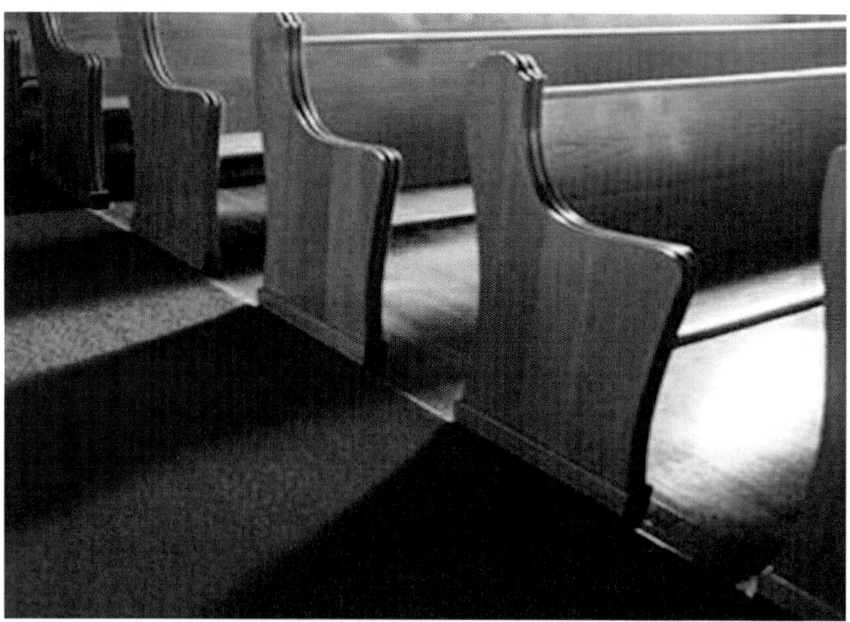

A Reason to Believe

Americans are one of the most religious people in the western world. And with good reason. In the United States, attending religious services at least once a week is a strong predictor of happiness.

A 2006 report by the Pew Research Center found that 43 percent of people who attend church at least once a week reported being "very happy" while only 26 percent of those who attend "seldom or never" said the same.

It doesn't matter which faith you profess. The key is regular attendance.

Why should being religious bring us so much happiness?

"Religious communities provide people with opportunities to support others in need," says Harold G. Koenig, M.D. professor of psychiatry and behavioral sciences at Duke University. "Contributing to the lives of others provides a deep sense of happiness and joy. If you can relieve someone's pain or provide for some of their basic needs, it fills you with a feeling that's hard to replicate."

In addition, just about every major religion encourages us to take good care of our bodies. For instance, religious people are less likely to drink heavily or smoke, says Koenig.

As a result, religious people are healthier, and health is one of the biggest predictors of happiness.

4 of 10
< Previous | Next >

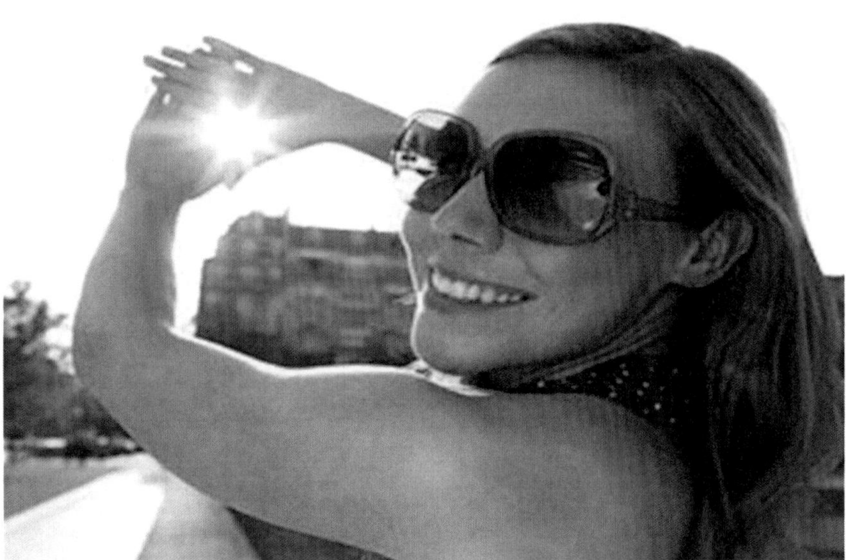

Let the Sunshine In

The region of the country you live in can impact your risk of suffering from depression—at least from November through April.

That's because those living in the northern part of the country are more at risk of suffering from seasonal affective disorder, a form of clinical depression brought on in the winter months by the shortening of the days and the later sunrise.

"In the United States, SAD is about five times more prevalent in the northern tier of states than in the far south," says Dr. Michael Terman, director of the Center for Light Treatment and Biological Rhythms at the Columbia University Medical Center.

But SAD is just the tip of the iceberg, explains Terman. "Less severe 'winter doldrums' occur at least three times more frequently than winter depression. Even more people experience one or more symptoms of winter depression—such as overeating or oversleeping—even though their mood stays under control."

Whatever the degree of impairment, symptoms tend to resolve in the spring. "Certainly there is no lack of happiness up north for the six months from May to October," Terman says.

How sunny is your city?

The NOAA has ranked cities according to the percentage of daylight hours when the sun is actually shining. While the length of winter days and the time of winter sunrise are the factors related to SAD, the sunnier cities do tend to be clustered in the South.

Sunniest big cities: Las Vegas (85 percent); Phoenix (85 percent); Sacramento, Calif. (78 percent); Los Angeles (73 percent); Miami (70 percent)

Darkest big cities: Seattle (43 percent); Pittsburgh (45 percent); Portland, Ore. (48 percent); Buffalo, N.Y. (48 percent); Cleveland (49 percent)

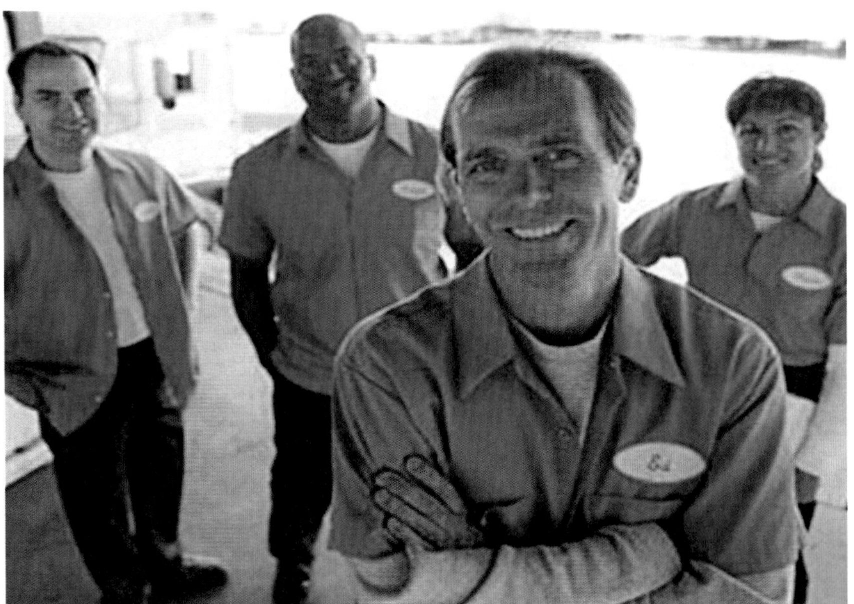

He Works Hard for His Happiness

Does working make you unhappy or happy? The answer: It depends. Toiling away at a job you hate may eat away at your happiness over time. But overall, being unemployed is worse for your state of mind than being employed—at least, that is, if you're a guy.

The Pew Research Center found that the percentage of men who said they were "very happy" was significantly lower for unemployed men (16 percent) than for employed men (37 percent). Unemployment had little impact on women's happiness.

The Pew researchers speculate that this is because more women than men are unemployed by choice, although the study didn't attempt to piece apart that difference.

Chris Peterson, a happiness researcher at the University of Michigan, suspects there are other factors at play as well. "Other studies have found that if a man loses his job, it can have both short-term and long-term psychological effects, even if he finds another job with equal salary," he says. "For women it's not unemployment that leads to unhappiness, but divorce."

In addition, Peterson stresses that money matters less than you'd think. "The engaged custodian is more likely to be happy than the independently wealthy, unengaged millionaire," he says. "We didn't evolve to be retired and sit on the couch."

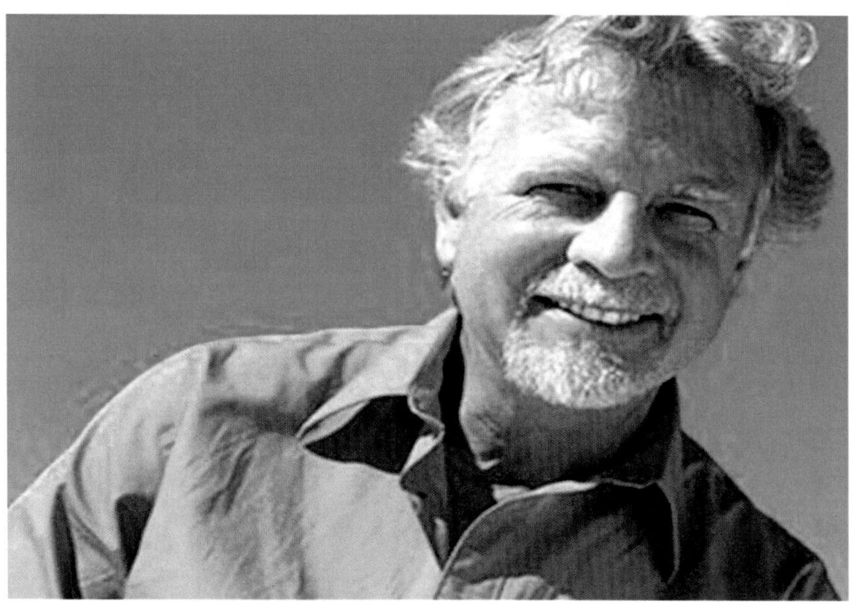

As Long As You Have Your Health

Perhaps it comes as no surprise to find that healthier people are happier than those who aren't as healthy. In fact, a 2006 report published by the Pew Research Center found that 48 percent of people who rated their health as "excellent" described themselves as "very happy," while only 15 percent of those who rated their health as "poor" said the same.

After all, it's harder to be happy when living with chronic pain or illness or when faced with a potentially life-threatening condition.

While health is strongly tied to happiness, lack of health is even more strongly correlated with lack of happiness. Of those who rated their health as "poor," a whopping 55 percent described themselves as "not too happy," while only 6 percent of those in "excellent" health said the same.

According to the Pew Research Center, health—along with religion and marriage—were among the strongest predictors of happiness, even when adjusting for a variety of other variables.

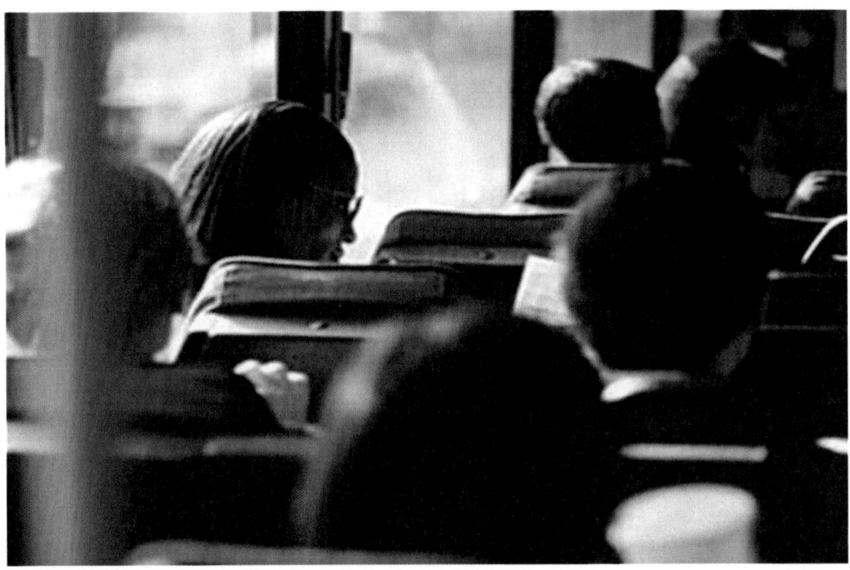

Time for Family, Friends, and Community

In the growing field of happiness research, one thing is overwhelmingly clear. People who are socially engaged are more likely to be happy—and less likely to be depressed—than those who aren't.

In fact, a 2005 *Time Magazine* poll found that the four most significant sources of happiness—children (77 percent), friendships (76 percent), contributing to the lives of others (75 percent), and spouse/partner (73 percent)—all involved spending meaningful time with other people.

The problem: "We're so caught up with extraordinary work burdens, we don't have time to enjoy the people we love or contribute to the lives of others," says Post.

That time crunch is quite real, says John de Graaf, president of the public policy organization Take Back Your Time. "Compared to thirty years ago, the average family now spends an extra 500 hours per year working outside the home."

We're also spending more time getting to work and back.

"Traffic is getting worse and we're not investing in mass transit," says de Graaf. "Most of the data I've seen shows that we've doubled our average commute times in the past generation."

Obviously, it depends on where you live—and where you work. Those most impacted: affluent families who chose even larger homes over living closer to work, and younger families who are priced out of homes of any size closer to centers of employment.

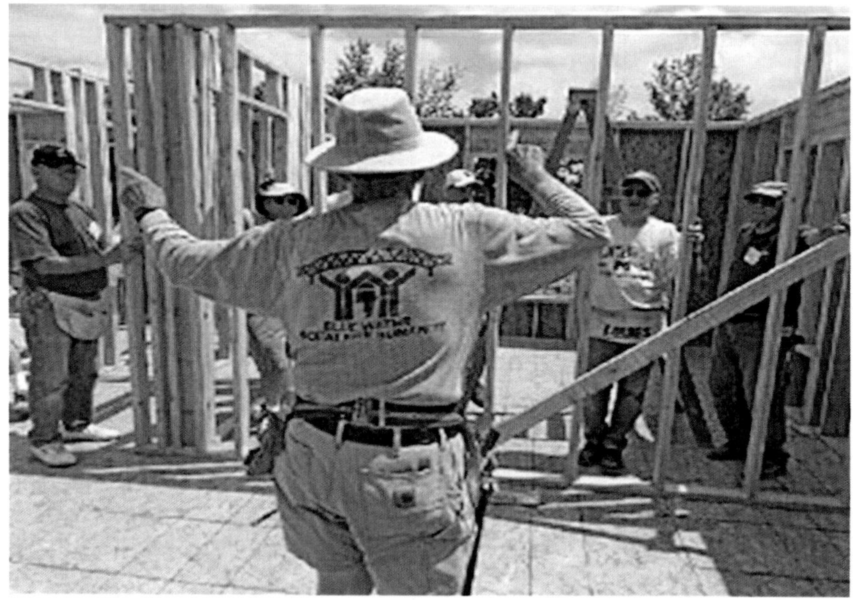

Giving for Your Own Good

This may come as a surprise to the "Me Generation," but happiness doesn't come from living in a big house, buying the latest techno-gadget, and getting stamps from exotic locales in your passport.

In fact, a 2005 poll by *Time Magazine* found that helping others was a major source of happiness for 75 percent of Americans.

"Volunteering is an opportunity to be socially engaged and contribute to the lives of others," says Stephen Post, a professor at Case Western Reserve University who co-authored the book,

Why Good Things Happen to Good People, with Jill Neimark. "It's not material goods that make us happy—it's having purpose and meaning in our lives."

In fact, some recent research suggests that we're actually hard-wired for helping. Even thinking about helping others is enough to stimulate the part of our brain associated with feel-good chemicals like oxytocin.

Helping others doesn't just make us happier, there's also evidence it makes us healthier, too. "Recent research out of England shows that cities with higher rates of volunteerism had the lower rates of depression and heart disease," says Post.

Don't have a lot of free time? No worries. People who volunteer just two hours per week (100 hours per year) enjoy lower rates of depression and better physical health.

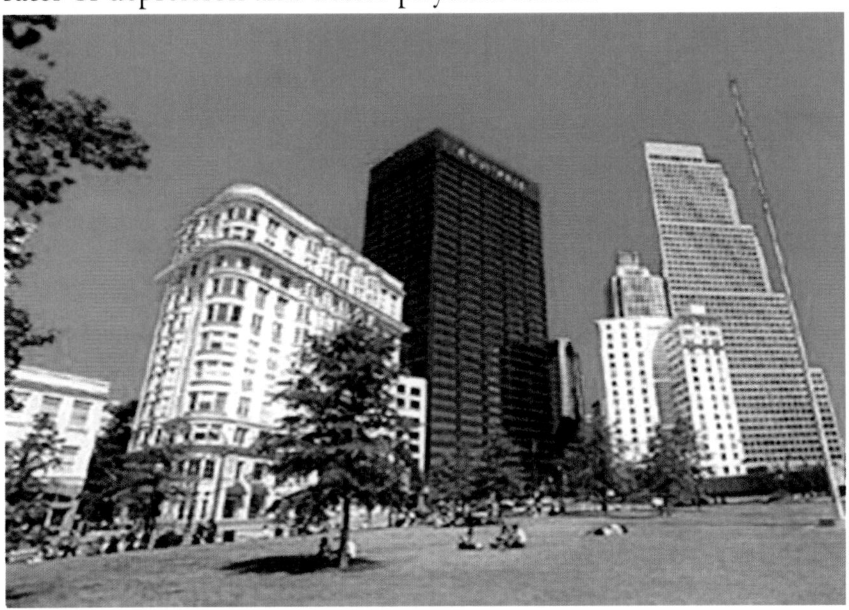

Good Urban Design

What does urban design have to do with happiness? More than you might think.

"The data strongly suggests that real community and real friendships are important keys to happiness," says Post. "Some cities make that possible in ways that others don't."

Post explains how urban design can facilitate social interaction—or work against it.

"Forty years ago, neighborhoods had sidewalks, front porches, and parks—geographical opportunities for people to be socially engaged," he says. "In many communities today, we are lacking these things. We don't know our neighbors anymore. We just get into our car pods and never see anyone. We no longer have the opportunity to stumble upon happiness by being good neighbors in our communities."

Good urban design and effective mass transportation can also determine how much time we spend commuting to work, and how much time we spend behind the wheel of a car running errands—both of which ultimately impact the amount of time we have for joyfully engaging with friends, family, and community.
msnbc.com staff and news service reports

Conclusion:

I have so much more to write but I must bring this book to an end.

I wish I could meet and talk with every person who reads this book, "The Naked Truth"; for I would encourage each of you to begin making lifestyle changes today-changes that will save you money, make you healthier, happier and more successful in everything you are striving to accomplish.

The eight laws of health that I have outlined and that the Weimar Institute penned the acronym NEWSTART to, are not new; they are as old as the bible itself, but are as fresh as the morning dew.

I have included a list of Lifestyle Teaching Centers that I highly recommend. Each one has varying lengths of programs from about a week up to a month. Some have live in programs.

Call the Lifestyle Teaching Center that is located nearest you and get started in putting your life back together.

I will be praying for each of you as you strive for excellence in an holistic approach to better living.

Appendix [Lifestyle Teaching Centers]

Uchee Pines Institute
30 Uchee Pines Rd
Seale, AL 36875-5702
334-855-4781
334-855-4765 Lifestyle Center

Weimar Institute
(20601 W. Paoli Lane)
PO Box 486
Weimar, CA 95736
916-637-4111
916-637-4408

Wildwood Lifestyle Center and Hospital
(1 Lifestyle Lane)
PO Box 129
Wildwood, GA 30757
706-820-1493
706-820-1474

Eden Valley Lifestyle Center
6263 NCR 29
Loveland, CO 80538
970-667-1770